ALLERGIES

NUTRITIONAL HEALTH SERIES

ALLERGIES

HOW YOUR DIET CAN HELP

Stephen Terrass

Thorsons
An Imprint of HarperCollins*Publishers*

Thorsons
An Imprint of HarperCollins*Publishers*
77–85 Fulham Palace Road,
Hammersmith, London W6 8JB
1160 Battery Street,
San Francisco, California 94111–1213

Published by Thorsons 1994

1 3 5 7 9 10 8 6 4 2

© Stephen Terrass 1994

Stephen Terrass asserts the moral right to
be identified as the author of this work

A catalogue record for this book is
available from the British Library

ISBN 0 7225 2984 8

Printed in Great Britain by
HarperCollinsManufacturing, Glasgow

CONTENTS

Dedication

This book is dedicated to Nicola, whose love, understanding, patience, encouragement and valuable input
have helped me immeasurably in the writing of this
manuscript.

ACKNOWLEDGEMENTS

The author wishes to thank the following for their valuable support and assistance in this project: Richard Passwater, Ph.D. for his inspiration, and for providing the foreword and reviewing the manuscript; editor Sarah Sutton and copy-editor Michele Turney; special thanks to Rand Skolnick, John Steenson, Cheryl Thallon and Leyanne Scharff for their valuable support; and Nibs Laskor for his help and generosity. Most of all, fondest thanks to Nicola Squire and Shirley Terrass for their love and encouragement.

This is an important book that could help thousands to understand and overcome allergies. It is estimated that at least 10 per cent of all patients seeking medical care do so because of allergies and food sensitivities. The figure would be much higher if more people realised that vague symptoms such as fatigue, headache, tension, sweating and bad breath are included among the symptoms of allergies. The most common cases are due to hay fever, and nearly half are due to food sensitivities. The remainder of the cases are due to inhaled or contacted substances or insect bites.

This book is based purely on scientific and medical research. Stephen Terrass has personal experience and enormous depth of knowledge of nutrition, which places him in a special position to unravel the scientific mysteries of allergies and to separate what works from what does not. A former allergy sufferer who found little relief via conventional medicine, Stephen Terrass has studied allergies in both Europe and the United States. He has helped countless allergy sufferers through his popular lectures and therapy sessions. Now this vast experience is being presented in book format for the first time.

Allergies supplies the reader with the necessary background information to help all understand, and it is done it in a manner that is simple to follow and exceptionally well organised. Using excellent analogies and understandable explanations, Stephen Terrass guides you through the maze of elimination diets, rotation diets and other methods of diagnosis testing. He takes you step by step through the processes that will elucidate whether you have a conventional allergy, a food intolerance or a chemical sensitivity. He then explains how you can suppress the symptoms and discomfort, and then treat the condition itself by natural methods. Conventional therapies are discussed and explained as well.

As a nutritional biochemist, I feel that a particularly useful part of this book is the discussion of nutrients and herbs with respect to specific allergies. There is much valuable information given here that should be on one hand for reference even by those who are not afflicted by allergies. Stephen Terrass is a student of the scientific literature and knows the science of nutrition extremely well. The reader can be assured that the advice given in this book has been proven by experience and is based on solid science.

Richard A. Passwater, Ph.D.
December 1993

Even if you lead the healthiest of lifestyles you can suffer from allergies. Perhaps, for no obvious reason, you feel generally unwell. Do you feel exhausted or sleepy after eating, or even all of the time? Maybe you suffer from chronic skin problems although you never eat junk food. You might have terrible bloating, gas or indigestion after every meal or, even stranger, only after breakfast. You might use the best and most expensive cosmetics, and yet still get persistent dark circles under the eyes. Perhaps you get frequent headaches or are depressed all the time for some unexplained reason. You may even be one of those unfortunate people who suffer from asthma or hay fever.

Allergy sufferers may visit seemingly every doctor listed in the phone book and never get a clear diagnosis. The reply sounds like a broken record: 'I am very sorry madam/sir, but there is nothing wrong with you.' Easy for them to say! They obviously do not spend half the day having a two-way conversation with their stomach, nor do they have to take their pyjamas to work with them to prepare for the uncontrollable urge to sleep that hits around 2 p.m.

When an allergy is identified as the problem, the sufferer generally feels very relieved. Even if the precise nature of the allergy is still to be discovered – what the person is allergic to – the initial diagnosis marks the end of a long road of uncertainty, and of being labelled a 'hypochondriac'.

It might seem strange to have symptoms such as headaches, digestive disturbances, depression, and dark circles under the eyes diagnosed as being caused by allergies. For this reason, many sufferers are sometimes just as disbelieving as those sceptics who call them a hypochondriac. However, if they are lucky enough to find out what they happen to be allergic to, and learn what to do about it, they quickly become aware that the rather strange diagnosis was perhaps the only correct one they have ever had.

UNDERSTANDING ALLERGIES

Recently there has been much publicity about the existence of allergy-related problems. This, in itself, is no great revelation, as we have known of the existence of allergies for years. What *is* of interest to the medical researchers are the specific mechanisms behind allergic reactions; the diversity and scope of what can produce an allergy, as well as the range of symptoms that can be scientifically connected to allergies. These aspects are being studied intensively. Many of the results of such research have been published in respected medical and scientific journals. Each new entry of information reveals another piece to the puzzle and further shows the need to continue to unravel the mystery behind allergies.

Why should we emphasise allergies so much in research? Allergies involve more than just sneezing when spring arrives or when a cat walks into a room. They are quite involved and intricate and indeed fascinating in the way they occur and develop. The more we know about allergies, the easier it becomes to help the sufferer, and to convince the sceptic (often the doctor) that the problem is real.

Another good reason for an increased understanding of allergies is the fact that the problem is much more common than we might assume. At the moment it is not possible to produce an accurate figure when assessing how many people suffer from allergies, particularly to foods, because most cases, sadly, still go undiagnosed. Statistics have been analysed in more definitive allergic cases. It has been suggested, for instance, that asthma, a potentially dangerous allergic condition, affects about three per cent of the United States population. It is likely to be about the same in countries with a similar diet, lifestyle, and/or climate.

We are all capable of developing an allergy to some or even many substances at any point in our lives. Just because you have lived 20 or 30 years without allergies does not mean that you will never suffer from them. (You may in fact have had allergies to many things all along without realising it as you have attributed the symptoms to something else.) Even more distressing is the huge range of substances that can cause an allergic reaction – literally hundreds – many of which we come into contact with every day.

Perhaps one of the most important reasons for an increased understanding of allergies stems from the incredible scope of the damage that they can do to a person, both physically and emotionally. The damage is not limited merely to the symptoms themselves, there is also a possibility of complications caused by the allergy itself, which can range from mild to quite severe.

SELF-HELP STRATEGIES

Regardless of the science behind allergies, most people simply want to feel better. Since there is frequently no proper diagnosis in such cases, it is important for people to be able to determine whether their symptoms are caused by allergies, what they are allergic to, and what they can do to relieve the symptoms and prevent the same reaction in the future.

This book will explain the mystery of allergies and how they relate to your physical and mental health. You will learn about the different types of allergies and their symptoms, what causes them, and how to find out what you are allergic to. You will find out how allergies can be treated and even prevented using safe, natural, and scientifically researched therapies such as vitamins and minerals, herbal medicine, and other natural substances as well as dietary management. If you feel that allergies may be your problem, relief may be on its way.

PLEASE NOTE: All of the information in these sections is based on published medical and scientific research and utilises safe, natural methods of therapy with almost no risks of side effects. Regardless of the safety, it is important to consult a qualified medical health practitioner before beginning any new health regime.

This book is not intended to be prescriptive, and should not be considered a substitute for proper medical advice in the event of a health problem. Whilst all efforts are made to ensure accuracy of the information, neither the author nor the publisher can accept legal responsibility for experimentation with the information discussed in this book.

CHAPTER 1

What is an Allergy?

The term 'allergy' is familiar to us all, yet the context in which it is typically used is so general that very few people actually know exactly what the word means. When we think of an allergy or an allergic reaction what usually springs to mind is a person sneezing, nose running and eyes watering, as a result of coming into contact with something he or she is allergic to. Perhaps this is because we are all aware of the relentless symptoms of hay fever or an allergy to dust or pet dander. These type of reactions are certainly the result of allergies, but allergies are definitely not limited to pollen, dust or animal dander.

Humans are capable of being allergic to literally thousands of things that they come in contact with at one time or another. Some of the more common allergens, which will be discussed later, include:

SEASONAL
- tree pollen
- grass pollen
- various spores

DOMESTIC
- dander from animal hair
- dust mites
- moulds

FOODS

- dairy products
- wheat
- corn
- citrus fruit
- shellfish
- eggs

Not only is the range of potential allergens quite vast, the range of allergic symptoms is certainly not limited to sneezing, watery eyes and runny nose. Some of the possible symptoms, which will also be discussed later, include:

- headache
- skin rash or irritation
- sneezing
- watery eyes
- runny nose
- respiratory congestion
- inflammation
- urticaria (hives)
- fatigue
- arthritis
- abdominal bloating
- indigestion and/or gas
- asthma
- depression
- catarrh
- chronic diarrhoea

People often wonder why a normal substance, such as a particular food, should cause an allergic reaction. We might be able to formulate an explanation if the food in question were inherently harmful, such as junk food; but this would not explain why 'healthy' foods, such as whole-wheat bread or fish, should cause an allergic reaction in some people.

THE COMMON DEFINITION

The common definition of an allergy is an abnormal sensitivity to a substance which brings about an adverse reaction. By abnormal, it is meant that the majority of people would not be likely to react similarly to such a substance. This definition seems very logical and understandable at face value, but it does not really begin to explain how or why the person is reacting abnormally to the substance in the first place. Unfortunately, it also does not represent the *proper* clinical definition of an allergy.

There are many different physiological reasons, besides an actual allergy, why a person may have an adverse reaction to a substance. When such reactions are being explained, however, they are generally grouped together with allergic reactions to simplify matters. Such reactions which are not related to allergies will briefly be discussed later. Such a generic use of the term allergy is not very helpful for people trying to get to the bottom of their particular problem if they suffer from unexplained reactions. While there are very advanced methods for properly diagnosing allergies (see Chapter 4), non-allergic reactions will not be accounted for on even the most accurate allergy tests. The problem this presents is quite substantial. Such diagnostic measures not only tell you whether or not you have allergies, they also detect what you are allergic to. If a test shows you are not allergic, then you are back to square one, perhaps feeling more desperate than ever because you are still unwell and do not know what is causing it. This is why one should be aware of the limitations to the most accepted definition of an allergy. After all, if you knew the proper categories of such reactions then you would not give up if an allergy diagnosis proved negative.

THE PROPER DEFINITION

So what is the most accurate definition of what an allergy involves? What distinguishes an allergy from any non-allergic reaction? You could quiz hundreds of qualified experts and perhaps come up with no clear consensus, but you would probably find a 'middle ground' in their replies similar to the common definition discussed above. As you know, this definition certainly has its limitations.

Fortunately, some substantial light has been shed on the issue by the Academy of Allergy and Immunology in the United States. Their interpretation has been adopted as the proper definition by many of the most respected experts in the fields of medicine, and it is this definition that will be used in this book when referring to allergies, particularly as they apply to foods.

The definition basically states that an allergy to a substance (such as in a food) involves an adverse reaction to a substance caused by an abnormal sensitivity which brings about an immune-related response by the body.

There is not much difference between this definition and the one mentioned previously, with the exception of the last part. Immune response refers to a function of your body's natural defence system. This specific relationship will be discussed shortly.

NON-ALLERGIC REACTIONS

These reactions, which are not related to the immune system, fall into different classes. It is helpful here to examine two of the main ones.

Intolerance

An intolerance generally involves foods or food additives (i.e. substances listed with E and a number after it on a food label). The clinical definition of an intolerance where it relates to food or food additives refers to an adverse reaction to a substance consumed which does not appear to mobilise the immune system. There are many different causes of intolerances which are not allergy related. A few of the more common are:

- an increased sensitivity to a particular chemical in the food (e.g. a toxic reaction to caffeine in chocolate or toxic agents found in certain under-cooked beans)
- difficulty digesting the food in question (due to lack of necessary enzymes)
- difficulty metabolising constituents of certain foods which are present in very large quantities (common in highly fatty foods)

Sensitivity

This can relate to foods, food additives and chemicals. Where it relates to foods, it represents a generic classification for any chronic adverse response to a food, whether allergic or non-allergic in nature. People who react in various adverse ways to exposure to a particular chemical are known as 'chemically sensitive'. These individuals can be sensitive to one or many different chemicals through contact by inhalation or skin, or in the case of chemical food additives, through oral ingestion. Chemicals that cause sensitivities in susceptible people are often inherently harmful to all people, but not normally in the doses involved in causing the reaction. The sensitivity can be due to many factors including:

- chronic over-exposure in the past
- liver disorders or weakness (common in alcoholism)
- excessive proneness caused by various physiological disorders
- repeated injury, trauma or lesions to an area physically exposed to chemical (either causing large amounts of chemical to enter the blood stream easily, or causing an increased local reaction to already weakened skin or perhaps respiratory or digestive tract)

Some of the more common offenders in chemical sensitivities include:

- formaldehyde
- food additives
- colours (e.g. tartrazine)
- flavours (e.g. monosodium glutamate)
- preservatives, (e.g. sulphur dioxide)
- synthetic dyes (e.g. in new clothing or carpet)
- diesel fumes
- natural gas

There are two main reasons why it is helpful to know the difference between an allergy and an intolerance or chemical-type sensitivity:

1 the treatment involved is often entirely different

2 it is important to know whether you are atopic (prone to allergy-related problems) so that you can take measures to reduce this tendency

In the case of true allergic reactions, the most effective treatment may centre on four main areas:

- avoiding the allergen (substance causing the allergic reaction)
- reducing the person's proneness to allergies
- strengthening the area prone to the allergy manifestation
- directly treating the symptoms

In intolerances and chemical sensitivities the treatment may centre on the following areas:

- avoiding the offending substance
- strengthening the area prone to irritation
- detoxifying the offending substance if necessary
- directly treating the symptoms

The difference between these two categories may seem slight, but the opposite is true. If you are allergic and do not know it, you may follow all the treatment areas applicable to intolerances and chemical sensitivities; and while you will improve, perhaps greatly, you are still as allergic as when you started. Even if you have strengthened the area which is usually affected by the reaction, that does not necessarily make you less allergic *per se*, although it will make you less prone to a reaction in that area. Allergic or atopic people frequently notice an ever expanding range of reactive areas in the body over time.

Being aware of some of the other factors known to

cause adverse reactions is not only useful to enable some people to identify possible irritants that they might not otherwise suspect, it also can be quite important to be aware of these in case you have been diagnosed as not showing any true allergies. It must also be kept in mind that chronic exposure to any substance to which you happen to be sensitive or intolerant can be both physically and emotionally detrimental beyond just the symptoms that the problem produces. This is true to varying degrees depending on both the substance and the person involved.

Sensitivities related to the above substances are generally not linked directly to an associated immune response, and thus would not be classified as allergies. Because of this, the most accurate tests for determining allergies would not account for these sensitivities. It is therefore very important to try to find a practitioner who is familiar with this area if it turns out that *allergies* are not your problem.

THE IMMUNE SYSTEM

In order to understand completely the causes and mechanisms behind allergies, we must first look at the factor that distinguishes them from other types of adverse reactions to particular substances – the immune system.

The human immune system is perhaps the most fascinating of all the body's functions. It is also, not surprisingly, among the most complex. The immune system has an immense responsibility – it carries out the process of keeping the body protected from disease and invasion by harmful substances. It is also responsible for making sure that only what belongs in the body stays in the body.

If you did not have a properly functioning immune system you would not be able to protect yourself from destructive forces such as cancer cells, viruses and harmful bacteria. This essential immune response is carried out by a 'military process' which runs 24 hours a day, 7 days a week, for your entire life. Now, for a military action you need an army, ammunition, instructions, and an enemy. An enemy is no problem. Your body is constantly full of cancer cells, harmful bacteria and viruses. Fortunately, your immune system normally has a large enough army, plenty of guns, bombs and bullets, and a well-organised plan. Your immune army is made up of many different forces. The main headquarters is found in the thymus gland behind your breastbone and in the bone marrow. This headquarters creates and houses many of the white blood cells, the primary fighting forces of the immune system.

At this point, you may be asking yourself a few questions. What actually is the connection between the immune system and allergies? Surely the immune system just destroys invaders such as cancer cells, harmful bacteria, viruses and anything that does not belong where it is in the body? Certainly cat fur, or perhaps wheat, are not going to enter a person's body and give them cancer or the flu, are they? So why would the immune system have anything to do with producing an allergy to them?

It is true that dust, pollen, and perhaps wheat and oranges, do not directly produce something the white blood cells are generally trained to destroy. Even substances that may contain harmful bacteria or are known to contain materials which promote cancer growth would only signal a normal immune response – not to the substance itself, but directly to the bacteria or to the cancer cells and only once they had developed.

At any rate, the immune system does not know of all of this confusion, nor does it care! It is not the immune system's job to ask questions. It has been given a responsibility to destroy any substance that does not belong where it is, or is perceived to be a foreign and potentially harmful invader, and any defective cell.

The cause of the allergy stems from the fact that the immune system does not recognise the allergy-causing substance (also known as an antigen) as something which belongs where it is and thus treats it as it does any other invader. The immune system may attack the allergen dieectly in the larger blood vessels or in the tissues. The manifestation of the allergic reaction will typically occur in the general location where the immune system attacks the allergen.

This is where the explanation becomes a bit difficult. Surely if wheat, or perhaps tree pollen, are considered invaders in one human's body, they would be considered an invader in any human's body. We all eat whole-wheat bread, for instance, in the same way. It goes through the body in the same way, and we digest and eliminate it in the same process. So what is the problem? The answer is rather complex, but in order to simplify it we will look at it from the standpoint of the different classifications of allergens. First we will look at food allergies then we will cover seasonal and environmentally oriented respiratory allergies.

CHAPTER 2

What Causes Allergies?

FOOD ALLERGIES

How an apparently non-threatening substance can provoke a reaction from the immune system that causes an allergy depends to a great extent on what the substance is. During digestion, foods are broken down into vital nutrients (proteins, fats, carbohydrates, vitamins, minerals, etc.).

The digestive system in which this process takes place is made up of many parts; the main ones are the mouth, the stomach and the intestines. Most of the breakdown of solid foods occurs as the result of digestive enzymes which are secreted by different parts of the digestive system (see Figure 1).

Once the macro-nutrients (proteins, fats and carbohydrates) are separated from the solid foods by digestion they are getting close to the point of being absorbed, primarily through the walls of the intestines. This way they can, depending on the nutrient, immediately or eventually enter the bloodstream where they can be transported throughout the body to sustain life. The proteins, carbohydrates and fats are only intended, however, to enter the bloodstream in their usable form. Protein is usable in the form of amino acids, carbohydrates as simple sugars, and fats as fatty acids. Figure 2 shows which digestive enzymes are primarily responsible for breaking down each nutrient.

Once the body has successfully broken down the macro-nutrients, the resulting substances are generally unable to present an allergy-related problem to the body. This seems to occur only when the macro-

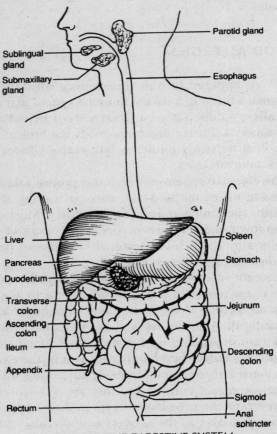

Figure 1. THE DIGESTIVE SYSTEM.

PART OF BODY	ENZYME(S)/ DIGESTIVE AGENT	SUBSTANCE DIGESTED
Mouth	Ptyalin	Carbohydrate/starch
Stomach	Hydrochloric acid	Proteins
	Pepsin	Proteins
	Gastric lipase	Fats
Duodenum	Amylase,	Carbohydrate/starch
	Lipase and	Fats
	Protease	
	(from pancreas)	Proteins
	Bile (from gall	
	bladder)	Fats
Intestines	Lactobacillus and	Sugars, yeast
(beyond	bifidobacterium	Bacteria
duodenum)		

Figure 2. DIGESTIVE ENZYMES.

nutrients, such as proteins or carbohydrates, are not completely broken down before they have the opportunity to absorb through the intestinal walls. It is at this point that a true allergic reaction to food can take place. This is the most common with food proteins. If, for example, a protein such as gluten (derived from wheat and certain other grains) is not adequately digested into free amino acids and remains as a protein when it is somehow absorbed through the intestinal wall, then it is capable of producing a reaction.

The white blood cells are accustomed to the entry of amino acids into the bloodstream from the moment of conception, and thus amino acids are not treated as invaders. The same thing could be said for simple sugars. Take as an analogy a man approaching a security point. If the guard has seen the same man pass that point several times before, the guard will allow him to pass every time. If that same person wears a disguise the next time, he will not gain entry by the same guard because he would not be recognised. If he then forces his way through the point, he will be attacked by all of the guards.

This is much the same as what occurs in the absorption of food nutrients. Amino acids and simple sugars are recognisable and thus gain free entry, but proteins and carbohydrates are not intended by the laws of human physiology to gain entry through the intestinal wall and subsequently into the bloodstream. If they somehow force their way through the security checkpoint at the wall, then they will be attacked by the white blood cells of the immune system.

How Food Allergens Absorb

It is now clear that absorption of whole macro-nutrients is not intended to occur. So how and why does it happen in the first place?

There are two main factors which allow for such a thing to happen. As a point of reference, we will look specifically at the enzymes which are associated with food proteins. One major problem is that the allergy sufferer may have a deficiency in the enzymes needed to digest proteins. A lack of hydrochloric acid or pepsin in the stomach or perhaps inadequate production of the protease enzymes from the pancreas is enough to cause an abundance of food derived proteins which will not be adequately digested.

There are many potential causes for deficiencies in protein-digesting enzymes. Enzymes have to be made and released by the body at the appropriate time and in the correct amounts to carry out their intended job. If the release of protein digesting enzymes is faulty either in the stomach or the pancreas then this must be dealt with. Often this problem is linked to one or more vitamin or mineral deficiencies (see Chapter 5).

If the problem is not linked to the release mechanism then it indicates a direct deficiency. Many people have a reduced ability to produce enzymes either in the stomach or the pancreas. This is also often linked to certain vitamin and mineral imbalances. Age, too, plays a strong role in this, especially in women. It has been determined that a very large percentage of women beyond their 40s have significant deficiencies in hydrochloric acid, the main protein-digesting enzyme. Age-linked digestive difficulties can also be very common in babies or very young children, who have yet to develop a completely efficient digestive ability towards as many food types as adults.

A deficiency in protein-digesting enzymes does not occur at some medically set range. A deficiency refers to when the available quantity is less than that which is required to deal with the amount of proteins being consumed. In other words, some people who suffer with food allergies consume excessive quantities of food-derived proteins which seems to make the body much less efficient at fully breaking down the load being presented to it. This is especially true of cereal proteins such as gluten which are notoriously difficult to digest completely. It is also more common when the same type of food protein (i.e. gluten) is being consumed repeatedly and/or in large quantities over a period of time.

It is a common phenomenon for people to develop an allergy to a food that previously gave them no problems, even for many years. Often in these cases you will find that they have much more frequently or repeatedly consumed the food, perhaps in large quantities shortly before the first allergic manifestation. This type of occurrence is often called a cyclic allergy.

Perhaps the major concern related to the incomplete breakdown of macro-nutrients stems from the fact that if a person fails to digest proteins into free amino acids, then he or she effectively becomes deficient in many individual essential amino acids. This can have far greater implications than the allergy itself.

Stress-linked Food Allergies

Stress can play a key role in almost every health disorder and allergies are certainly no exception. The effect stress has on digestion has been well-documented. In the early stages of stress the hormone adrenaline is released. Among other effects, adrenaline-release signals a shunting of blood away from the digestive system, leading to a slowing or shutting down of the digestive process. If stress is a chronic problem, digestion may frequently be virtually non-functional. This, in itself, is not the end of the world, but it does become a major problem if the individual happens to have eaten during or soon before the onset of the stress. If he or she frequently eats during this period of time, then the problem of inadequate protein or carbohydrate digestion will be particularly likely. The obvious rule here would be to avoid eating when under stress. As we all well know, however, this is easier said than done, as one of the favoured methods of comforting ourselves during stress is eating!

Bowel Permeability

The question is frequently asked, 'A lot of people eat large amounts of foods that are high in protein or carbohydrate, probably far in excess of what their digestive enzyme production can handle, so why don't more people suffer with food allergies?' There are two answers to this question. The first is that many more people have food allergies than know they do. The second answer has to do with the bowel.

Perhaps the most telling factor in the development of food allergies is the state of the bowel. While it is certainly the case that a person must first incompletely break down food components before an allergy can occur, it is clear that this is not all that uncommon in people without known allergies. The missing piece to this puzzle is a little known factor called excessive bowel permeability.

The intestinal wall is designed to act like a fine mesh sieve, letting through necessary substances and keeping out others. Only micro-nutrients and water are supposed to be able to get through this wall. The micro-nutrients (including vitamins, minerals, amino acids, fatty acids and simple sugars) are small enough to fit through, at least this is the case when the intestinal wall is healthy.

Unfortunately there are frequently cases where a person's intestinal wall has, for one reason or another, an altered texture or integrity. Some more common alterations in the bowel include:

- intestinal injury or lesions (e.g. Crohn's disease)
- inflammation of intestinal wall
- bacterial imbalances in the intestines
- infantile permeability from incomplete development of digestive system

Some more common causes of these alterations include:

- improper digestion
- chronic constipation or diarrhoea
- overgrowth of the yeast *Candida albicans*
- bacterial imbalances in the intestines
- chronic laxative use
- chronic antacid use
- chronic antibiotic use
- chronic steroid use
- alcohol abuse

In many cases, the integrity of the intestinal wall can be significantly weakened to the extent that the once tight barrier becomes more porous. Larger molecules such as those of incompletely digested proteins can then go through the wall to gain entry into the bloodstream. It is these large molecules that become antigens, the specific agents to which the antibodies of the immune system bond before the other white blood cells attack. The first symptomatic manifestation of the food allergy can occur at this point of the intestinal wall, or elsewhere in the body. In order for a symptom to occur locally, at the intestinal wall, there would usually be some type of inflammation, irritation or lesion. One reason for this is that in such cases, there are likely to be large amounts of various white blood cells available.

If you think you have a reason to be disappointed if a tea bag lets through lots of sediment into your drink, then you should be absolutely livid when your intestinal wall allows things into your bloodstream that are not supposed to get through. The bowel permeability problem can start a cycle of deterioration. The allergy reaction caused, in part, by the bowel permeability may itself further harm the bowel integrity. This exacerbates the bowel permeability, which makes you more allergic, and so on

Clearly, the best way to prevent excessive bowel permeability is to avoid any of the common factors that would tend to precipitate alterations in the bowel tissue in the first place. This is not always possible, but there are natural methods that can help correct some of these factors (see Chapter 5).

Genetic Tendency

There clearly seem to be a greatly increased tendency to food allergies in people whose parents have had a history of them. Research has revealed that when one of the parents has suffered with the problem, about one in three of their children will be allergic. If both parents were food allergic, then approximately two out of three of their children would be allergic. There are different opinions as to why this might be the case, but what is clear is that:

1 There is a proven genetic link in cases of diseases that can injure the bowel integrity (e.g. Crohn's disease).
2 There are obvious similarities in the eating habits of parents and their children (same foods eaten in similar quantities and similar frequency).
3 It is possible for certain immune-related factors to be genetically passed on.
4 Stress-related factors may be similar.

There are other possibilities as well, but these are some of the more likely. There may well be a familial tendency toward allergies of various types. People with a general tendency towards allergy-induced symptoms and disorders are sometimes classified as being atopic.

Common Allergy-causing Foods

As we have seen, starches and other food constituents can cause allergic reaction as well. Literally hundreds of different foods could be implicated in allergies. The shocking truth is that it is perhaps more common for a person to be allergic to several foods rather than to just one.

For possible food-allergy sufferers, it is important to be aware of the more common allergy-producing foods so that they can better assess their diet. Included among the more common allergy producing foods are:

- dairy products
- wheat
- corn
- citrus fruits
- eggs
- yeast
- peanuts
- fish
- shellfish
- oats
- rye
- barley
- beef
- chicken

There are many others as well, but these are frequently noted to be a problem.

The above list excludes a wide variety of foods, drinks and ingredients which are known to produce allergy-like or pseudo-allergic reactions; in other words, reactions that are not mediated by the immune system and antibody binding, but are adverse reactions nonetheless. A common sample includes:

- chocolate
- alcohol
- strawberries
- cured meats (bacon, sausage)
- tea
- coffee
- sugar
- tartrazine (food colouring)
- sulphur dioxide (food preservative-common in dried fruits)

People *are* capable of being allergic to many things in this classification as well, but the reactions are perhaps more common in the intolerance or chemical-sensitivity category.

Allergies or intolerances to the foods or beverages in the two above lists can occur in any combination. Remember that what a person is allergic to can be *any* food imaginable. Some allergy-causing foods are quite obscure. Bear in mind that you are probably much more likely to be allergic to something you consume frequently and perhaps in large quantities. What constitutes 'frequently' or 'large quantities' depends on both the person and the food involved.

RESPIRATORY AND SEASONAL ALLERGIES

Not all respiratory symptoms of allergies are caused by a respiratory or inhaled allergen. As a matter of fact, one of the most common symptoms of food allergies is respiratory congestion. Once it enters the blood system, the food-derived antigen can travel to many different places where it can produce symptoms. If the antigen happens to settle in the location of respiratory membranes then the usual response is an over-production of mucus leading to sinus or lung congestion.

There are different classifications of respiratory-type allergies and non-allergic respiratory reactions. Some are linked to ingested food antigens or ingested substances or chemicals (especially preservatives such as sulphur dioxide and sulphites). Others are linked directly to inhaled antigens or chemicals.

The most common examples of respiratory-type reactions are asthma and seasonal allergies such as hay fever. In the case of hay fever, the reaction is related to a specific allergen being inhaled. With asthma the reaction can either be brought about by an actual antigen or by a non-antigenic irritant.

The respiratory tract, including the oxygen-transporting tubes called bronchioles, the lungs and the sinuses play the major role in conditions such as asthma and hay fever. The tendency to such problems can be related to either an excessive sensitivity in the person's airways, an excessive exposure to irritants or antigens, or perhaps excessive levels of inflammatory chemicals near the surface tissue of the respiratory tract.

The excessive sensitivity could be caused by a weakness in the integrity of the lining of the respiratory tract. This can be very similar to excessive bowel permeability. Such a sensitivity can cause the respiratory walls to be more easily aggravated by a potential antigen, such as pollen; it can cause the walls to be more likely irritated by an inhaled chemical, such as cleaning solvents; and it can make the walls more vulnerable to inflammation.

When the reaction is caused by an allergic response to an inhaled antigen such as pollen, or an irritant such as a cleaning solvent, the reaction generally occurs fairly rapidly. In some cases of respiratory reaction to a food allergen, the symptoms can be either almost immediate or they can take a while to manifest.

Asthma

Asthma is one of the most distressing of all health disorders linked to allergies. A well-known condition, asthma is characterised by a release of thick mucus in the lungs, bronchial spasm, and an inflammatory constriction of the airways, all of which can restrict breathing. The extent to which the breathing is restricted varies from person to person and from occurrence to occurrence in the same person. In the milder cases, slight shortness of breath and minor wheezing may occur. In the more severe cases, however, breathing can be restricted to dangerous, even potentially fatal levels. It occurs more frequently in children before teenage years, and in this age group it is about twice as prevalent in boys. In adults there is not much difference in the prevalence between men and women. There are two main classifications of asthma.

INTRINSIC ASTHMA

Non-allergic asthma is linked to various factors which either may be irritating to the respiratory tract or cause mechanical asthmatic response. These factors may include:

- various inhaled fumes
- excessive exertion or exercise
- bronchitis or related illness
- stress
- excessively cold weather

- various airborne particles
- various food preservatives or additives

EXTRINSIC ASTHMA

Asthma related to true allergic response to an antigen which brings about respiratory reaction. Factors may include:

- tree or grass pollens
- spores or moulds
- dander

Because of the potential risks involved in asthma, it is vitally important to be able to distinguish what factor or factors are responsible for the problem. Once they have been identified, it is necessary to eliminate them as much as possible. Methods of reducing allergic tendencies as well as asthmatic symptoms and strengthening the airways will be discussed later (see Chapter 5).

Hay Fever

Many people think of hay fever as the classic example of an allergy. Perhaps this is because so many people actually suffer with the problem, generally at the same times.

Hay fever is a generic term which is used to describe the primarily seasonal reaction to pollens and spores. It is sometimes known as allergic rhinitis. Pollens from various trees are major contributors in the spring, and in the summer, weeds and various grasses are prominent. The pollens and spores that travel by air are inhaled by the hay fever sufferer and stimulate an immune-related antibody effect locally in the respiratory tract. The end result of this process is an inflammatory response, the all too familiar symptoms such as sneezing, watery eyes and runny nose.

There is likely to be a tendency in hay fever sufferers that makes them more likely to develop the problem. Other than being generally susceptible to allergies, there is probably going to be more of a local tissue weakness. There are many sufferers of quite severe food allergies who have never had hay fever. As you may guess, allergy symptoms are more likely to strike in the areas of the body that have the weakest tissues.

It is obviously not practical to avoid the allergen involved in hay fever, as it would require moving to an area virtually free of such allergens. Suffice it to say that there are ways of reducing the problem both symptomatically and in terms of susceptibility (see Chapter 5.)

CHAPTER 3

Allergy Symptoms

The list of potential allergy-related symptoms is quite immense, a fact that contributes to the erroneous opinion of some people that such sufferers are 'hypochondriacs'. Just as food-allergic people are more likely to have multiple food allergies than just one, people with allergies are also likely to have more than one symptom even if they are only allergic to one substance. Bearing this in mind, it seems a bit more understandable how a non-allergy sufferer could be sceptical. The published research shows, however, that diagnosed allergy sufferers have *real* symptoms which are *not* purely psychosomatic.

The problem is that once a sufferer has a consistent reaction to a particular food, he or she may develop a 'learned response' which would be difficult to eliminate even if the person consumed only negligible quantities of the offending food, far too little to produce a reaction under normal circumstances. It must be kept in mind, however, that some people are truly so sensitive that even a minute amount of an offending food can produce a *real* immunological response.

Some of the most common symptoms associated with allergies are as follows:

FOOD ALLERGIES
- headaches/migraine
- skin rash or irritation
- eczema
- urticaria (hives)
- fatigue
- depression
- abdominal bloating
- indigestion and/or gas
- dark circles under eyes
- inflammation
- dizziness
- sinus congestion/catarrh
- asthma
- arthritis
- diarrhoea

RESPIRATORY ALLERGIES (ASTHMA/HAY FEVER)
- wheezing
- laboured breathing
- thick, difficult-to-expectorate mucus
- coughing
- sneezing
- watery, itchy eyes
- runny, itchy nose

HOW THE SYMPTOMS OCCUR

In the case of allergies, once the antigen has passed the 'point of no return', antibodies (called immunoglobulins) are what start the unfortunate chain reaction. So how does this bonding of antigens with immunoglobulins bring about the symptoms? The answer depends greatly on the type of symptoms being produced, but for a point of reference, let us look at allergic reactions such as asthma, eczema and allergic arthritis.

All three conditions involve a reaction in various tissues in the body. All three also happen to be medically classed as inflammatory conditions – in other words, disorders where certain tissues are inflamed. Asthma, as mentioned before, involves irritation and eventual inflammation of the tissue in the walls of the airways, Eczema, a very common symptom of food-related allergies, is a condition where patches of skin become red, inflamed and eventually begin to weep. Arthritis is inflammation of the joint tissues.

There are two main processes involving immuno-globulins which may bring about allergy symptoms in not only these three cases but also many other allergic reactions. The process starts with the bonding of immunoglobulins with the antigen. In one very common scenario the process continues with the triggering of certain other white blood cells to seek, destroy and devour the antigen.

When the load of immune complexes (antigens bound to antibodies) is not too heavy, the white blood cells are relatively efficient at disposing of the 'cellular rubbish' left behind. If the load is heavy, perhaps due to large consumption of the antigen in a short period of time, then the residual immune complexes that are not immediately cleaned up can injure the tissue in the area. It is important here to note that foods containing substances called vaso-active amines (such as cheese and chocolate) may exacerbate this problem.

A slightly different, particularly disturbing, second phase may also arise. In more immediate reactions, the antigen may be bound to immunoglobulin IgE that is

already attached to a white blood cell called a mast cell.
Mast cells are responsible for releasing inflammation-
causing chemicals such as histamine and leukotrienes.
The antigen bonding may cause the release of large
amounts of these chemicals, thereby producing
significant local inflammation. This is very common in
asthma, eczema and arthritis.

Two other problems may arise in this second phase.
Sometimes inflammation and tissue irritation can occur
as a result of certain white blood cells attacking antigens
without the help of antibodies. Another possible reaction involves what is known as a cytotoxic effect. In this
situation, the antibody bonding initiates a process
where any cell which happens to be attached to the
antigen is destroyed.

Regardless of which second phase occurs, a typical
end result or third stage of the antigen pathway
involves an inflammatory response which may be
directly or indirectly responsible for many of the symptoms that occur. This can even be the case in symptoms
such as migraine headaches and diarrhoea as well as the
more logical connections, such as joint swelling, breathing
constriction or perhaps skin redness.

Whether the inflammatory response is immediate or
delayed, the release of histamines and the production of
leukotrienes are responsible. This should make even
more sense when you consider one of the primary classes of medication given for allergic symptoms such as
hay fever – antihistamines.

Some of the other, more common symptoms of allergies may be at least partly due to an direct association
with inflammation. This is primarily the case with food
allergies. Because we know that the first manifestation
of a food allergy (as opposed to a food intolerance) is

likely to occur at the intestinal barrier at the earliest, the intestinal wall itself is likely to pay a heavy price in a battle between the immune system and the antigen.

It is not unlike a real war where bombs are being dropped, gunfire is raging and tanks are rolling. In a real war, not only are men, buildings and planes destroyed or damaged, the land beneath them is plundered as well. When a war ensues between the antigen and the immune cells at the intestinal barrier, the surrounding tissue can be damaged by the fallout. The typical result is inflammation.

The inflammation of the intestinal wall can frequently occur at a site such as in the small intestine, where most nutrient absorption takes place. The change in the integrity of the small intestinal wall can cause malabsorption to occur, which means that absorption is reduced or hindered, perhaps quite significantly. A severe deficiency in essential nutrients may result, thus leading to a host of problems such as fatigue and depression. Another detrimental cycle can then occur. Many essential nutrients are capable of reducing allergic symptoms and even the tendency towards allergies in the first place. Deficiencies in these nutrients would, if anything, lead to increased allergic tendencies and symptoms.

CHAPTER 4

Diagnosing Allergies

This chapter concentrates, for the most part, on food allergies. This is because, when it comes to diagnosing environmental allergies and/or allergic reactions initiated in the respiratory tract, a do-it-yourself approach is not so appropriate. It is best, in such cases, to consult a qualified practitioner.

One of the problems with diagnosing allergies stems from the fact that it is so difficult to find a doctor who is willing to accept that your symptoms may be related to food allergies, and qualified to test for such a thing. The other problem stems from the impracticality, both logistic and financial, of having testing carried out by a doctor or practitioner. Although some *are* able to test for allergies, they are often not capable of adequately diagnosing in many cases of food intolerances.

ELIMINATION/REINTRODUCTION DIETS (CHALLENGE TESTING)

Fortunately there are methods of testing that do not require the services of a doctor or practitioner – and they are free of charge. The most suitable method of self-testing for the purpose of identifying offending foods is known as the elimination diet. Although elimination diets (also known as oligoantigenic diets) avoid the cost of practitioners and testing procedures, they do require a substantial investment in diligence, patience, discipline and monitoring. If the necessary effort is put into such a process, very impressive results can be achieved.

Unfortunately, no perfectly accurate, all-encompassing method of identifying food reactions as a whole is available. Some of the testing methods are very inaccurate, or at least their accuracy cannot yet be verified scientifically. Others are accurate to a point. The best are very accurate but have limitations on what they can determine. The elimination diet fits into this last category.

The Pros and Cons of the Elimination Diet

PROS

- no expense
- no practitioner or doctor required either to administer or assess results
- very good at helping identify almost any potentially offending food, whether due to allergy, intolerance, or chemical-type sensitivity
- very useful in determining which symptoms are associated with which foods

CONS

- requires dietary discipline, patience and monitoring
- it can take several weeks to get a more complete variety of foods tested
- not recommended in cases of food-induced severe breathing restriction or other severe anaphylactic reactions
- it does not determine whether reactions are due to allergies, intolerance or sensitivities

This diet is generally a very useful tool in your efforts to deal with food reactions of all types. In spite of the fact that it does not distinguish between allergies and intolerances, the first priority is to know what is causing the reaction and the subsequent symptoms so that the offending food(s) can be avoided. For this purpose, elimination diets are excellent.

How They Work

There are various methods of carrying out elimination diets, but here we will look at a classic example. The premise behind such a diet is that only a few specified foods may be eaten – all others must be eliminated.

Such a diet is known (perhaps not so fondly by the sufferer) as the 'lamb and pears diet' due to the inclusion of these foods on the permitted list. It consists of foods which are not typically known to be highly allergic. Conversely, the highly allergic foods such as milk, cheese, wheat, shellfish and eggs are absolutely forbidden.

When buying and/or preparing the foods which are allowable on this diet, it is important to make sure that they contain no ingredients, regardless of how small the quantity, which are not in the approved diet. This is especially a concern with buying prepared foods or eating out, so check labels and avoid restaurant sauces, dressings and such unless you can approve the ingredients first.

PLEASE NOTE: If any of your typical symptoms persist beyond a week or so of the elimination part of the diet, then it is very likely that you may be sensitive, allergic or otherwise, to something in the elimination diet. If this happens then the diet may have to be further restricted.

This rather simple diet is followed for anywhere between a week or two to a month. The reason for this time period is that it can take a while for the antigens that were ingested before the diet to be fully eliminated from the blood and tissues; it gives the immune system an opportunity to back down from its stage of 'red alert'; and it allows the tissues inflamed from the last bout with antigens to settle and heal somewhat. This process allows you, hopefully, to be symptom-free or relatively so by the time the trial period is over. Why? You need a 'clean slate' for diagnostic purposes because it is at this point that you being to reintroduce the eliminated foods one by one.

It is important that the reintroduction phase is taken a food at a time. If more were introduced at once, it would be impossible to know which food was responsible if a reaction occurred. In the more strict (and more accurate) form of this diet, only one type of food is reintroduced every couple of days. This allows for a delayed reaction. If a reaction is noted, then that food is often eliminated immediately. A couple of days after the first reintroduction, another food is introduced. This same process is carried out over and over until all the intended foods are checked. All reactions and associated symptoms should be recorded in terms of how they manifested, how severe they were, how long they took to occur, and how much of the food was consumed before the reaction first occurred. This will provide a helpful reference for the future.

Do not be surprised if the reactions you experience during the reintroduction phase are actually worse or more acute than before you did the elimination diet. It is common for a person to become even more sensitive to a food antigen after such a break from it. Although this can be uncomfortable, it certainly helps pinpoint specific reactions and symptoms, and also helps discipline the person to avoid the food in the future. This is especially important to use as a motivational tool because, as you will remember from earlier in the book, it is more common to develop an allergy to a food that you consume frequently and/or in large quantities, favourite foods, in other words. How would you feel if someone suggested that you should stop eating your favourite food? You might well laugh at them as you go on relishing that piece of pizza or bowl of chocolate ice cream. Now how would you feel about eliminating your favourite food or foods if you have proven to yourself that they are the real cause of your debilitating, nauseating, blinding two-day migraine headaches? Is it really worth spending five minutes eating that cheeseburger and twenty minutes with diarrhoea? At any rate, this type of elimination/reintroduction diet is frequently used to great effects provided the person has the forbearance to complete the process without 'cheating'.

Another type of elimination/reintroduction involves fasting for up to a week prior to a similar method of reintroduction. In this case, the term 'elimination diet' is no exaggeration. This type of diet is likely to be more accurate than the previously mentioned elimination diet, but cannot be recommended unless the person is under a doctor's supervision or is experienced in long-term fasting.

A Step-by-step Guide

STEP 1

Start a food diary. It is best to do this straight away in case you react to any of the allowable foods in the elimination phase. Keep a daily record of:

- foods that are allowed (see step 2)
- times of each meal
- approximate quantity of whichever food is being introduced on a particular day
- any reaction which occurs as a result
- approximately how long it took after ingestion for the reaction to occur
- whether the recorded reaction matches any chronic symptom which was experienced prior to the elimination diet

STEP 2

Eliminate all foods except for:

- lamb
- chicken*
- rice
- potatoes*
- broccoli**
- cauliflower**
- cooked cabbage**
- or similar vegetables**
- pears**
- apples**
- bottled or purified water
- apple or pear juice**

* Occasionally acceptable. Although not as common as allergies to dairy products, wheat, or citrus fruit, allergies to chicken or potatoes are not all that unusual either. A good rule with such marginal foods is to eliminate them from the allowable list if you normally eat them several times a week. Remember, allergies are more likely to develop to foods which are consumed very frequently.

** Preferably organic if available. Many people have a chemical sensitivity to various pesticides and other agricultural sprays used on commercial fruit and vegetables. Such sensitivities may produce symptoms that would make it difficult to judge accurately any reaction from a food being reintroduced.

STEP 3

Eat nothing but those foods on the allowable list for at least one week, up to one month if necessary. The duration is up to your discretion, but the longer you keep up the diet, the more accurate the reintroduction or challenge results are likely to be. Remember, it is important to adequately rid the body of antigenic contact, to let any affected body tissues heal and allow the immune system to settle.

STEP 4

After 1–4 weeks, reintroduce one food at a time for up to two days. If no reaction occurs move on to the next food for two days. If a reaction does occur discontinue the food immediately.

If a reaction occurs, it is often recommended to wait for a couple of days before testing the next food to allow the antigenic effect to run its course and be eliminated; this is particularly useful when the reaction does not occur until the second day of testing.

STEP 5

Repeat step 3 for all the foods you intend to test. Be thorough: if you want to test something new in the future, you will have to repeat the preliminary elimination diet again.

STEP 6

Assess the data you have collected and determine what foods should be in your new diet.

STEP 7

Avoid the offending foods for four to five months. After this period, you may choose to begin the organisation of a rotation diet.

> **CAUTION:** When a person is prone to severe constriction of the airways such as in severe asthma or another form of anaphylaxis (immediate, severe reaction), re-introduction/challenge testing can be dangerous. This is especially true since the person may react even more severely after the elimination phase than before it. As a result, such measures are not recommended in these cases.

ROTATION DIETS

Once you have identified the offending foods, the first goal is to eliminate or avoid them. Sometimes, in severe cases, it is even recommended that all foods belonging to the same food group as the food you are allergic to are avoided. After a while, perhaps two to four months depending on the person, many of the offending foods can be reintroduced *on an occasional basis,* e.g. once every four to seven days. These food produce what are known as cyclic allergies. Foods in the fixed allergy class will produce a reaction regardless of how long they have been avoided, and thus should never be eaten.

Cyclic food allergies begin after a period of frequent ingestion. Reintroducing a food that is causing such an allergy should be done through a rotation diet. The premise behind a rotation diet is that a cyclic allergy may be caused by exceeding a certain 'threshold' beyond which the immune system will react. As long as there is an adequate break between the times when the particular food is eaten, and the amounts consumed are not too much, the reaction does not occur.

A good analogy is a leak in the roof through which water is dripping. If you put a bucket underneath the leak, then it does not present a major problem until the bucket overflows, and as long as you keep emptying the bucket, it will not overflow. This bucket also gives you an opportunity to fix the roof! If you compare this to a cyclic food allergy, the antigen is the leak; the bucket is the leeway before your immune system acts; the overflow represents the reaction and the emptying of the bucket is what happens during the break from the food, and the longer the break, the more times the bucket is emptied. On the other hand, if the size of the hole in the roof increases, then the water begins to pour into the bucket and you may quickly have a disaster on your hands. By the same token, if you choose to eat vast amounts of the food you are rotating, then your proverbial bucket overflows rapidly and you are likely to have an allergic reaction again.

The typical rotation diet, which was created originally by Dr Herbert Rinkel in the 1930s, involves not only foods to which you are allergic, but also those to which you are not allergic. The point behind this is that atopic people are more prone to develop allergies to new foods if they eat them too often, so a rotation protects the person not only from recurrence of the old allergy symptoms but also any new developments. This is an even more sensible approach when you consider that when our diet is restricted, we tend to make the most of what we still *can* eat often with disastrous results. A vicious circle can creep in: the more new foods you become allergic to while trying to avoid your old allergies, the more you have to eat of the allowable foods just to take in ample nutrients and calories. Some allergy sufferers probably have nightmares that a time will come when they have nothing left to eat that they are not allergic to other than steamed turnips!

Even if you do not want to rotate your entire diet, it is vital that all reintroduced allergy foods are rotated. Remember that only cyclic allergy foods can be reintroduced into your normal diet. You can tell whether or not a food is causing a cyclic allergy by your reaction to it. If it is not cyclic you will react to it, probably even in small quantities, *whenever* you try to reintroduce it.

A good rotation diet simply involves eating each food at intervals of four days to a week or so. This would be the case whether rotating all foods or just those to which you are reacting at the time. It is important to keep a record of what you eat when, so that you rotate each food correctly.

A Step-by-step Guide

STEP 1
Start a daily food diary so that you can be certain what foods are allowable, and when. It can be planned as long in advance as is practical, but you may want to assess it occasionally to see whether it needs any adjustments.

STEP 2
If you are rotating only foods to which you are allergic, delegate a particular day for each of the offending foods you intend to reintroduce. How many different things

will be in a particular day's meals depends on your dietary preference. If you are rotating all foods, delegate a particular day for all food types being consumed. Once again, how many different things will be in a particular day's meals depends on your dietary preference. While it is not essential, rotating *all* foods is valuable in preventing allergies to new foods, as those who avoid allergy-causing foods tend to compensate by over-eating ones that they tolerate.

STEP 3

Once each food has been allocated a particular day in your organised plan, eat the foods on their first allocated days and do not eat them again for four to seven days or so. You may choose to judge which foods warrant a four-day cycle and which need a seven-day rest based on the severity of the allergic reaction. The more severe the allergy, the more rest required.

STEP 4

If reactions occur to any of the reintroduced foods, particularly if they do so immediately or in the very early stages of the rotation plan, then it can logically be assumed that these are fixed-allergy foods and must be avoided.

Once you have mastered the routine of either the elimination/introduction diet or the rotation diet – or both – it will make life much easier to tolerate. Not only will you find following the diet easier and less stressful, you will also start to gain control over your allergies. It is well worth the effort.

OTHER METHODS OF DIAGNOSIS TESTING

Laboratory testing methods are also available to the

allergy sufferer, which have certain advantages and disadvantages. At this point we will look briefly at some of the more easily available methods which do not involve special diets.

RAST (Radio Allergo Sorbent Test)

The RAST test is among the most suitable and accurate of all allergy-testing measures. A blood sample is taken, from which is calculated the extent of antibody production to food substances. The foods are tested separately, and the results can show not only what the person is allergic to but also, to an extent, the severity. The test is excellent for allergies but is not effective for non-allergic intolerance or food-chemical sensitivity. The test is very selective and is probably more likely to be accurate in immediate-reaction allergies.

The RAST test is relatively expensive, particularly if it involves testing for many different foods. On the positive side, it is neither uncomfortable nor time-consuming for the individual being tested.

Cytotoxic Test

This also involves taking a blood sample. This test looks at the way in which the appearance of the circulating white blood cells alters after exposure to antigens. Unfortunately, there is no exact standard for these alterations, so the assessment of the results is, to a great extent, up to the judgement of the person giving the test. This test is therefore somewhat limited in its accuracy compared to RAST testing. It is nevertheless a decent tool, especially as a confirmation of results of other testing methods, and it is not as expensive as a RAST test.

Pulse Test

The pulse test is one of the most simple and practical of all the tests. It is based on an observation by Dr Arthur Coca that the pulse rate of an allergic individual seemed to speed up significantly soon after ingesting a food to which he or she was allergic. Many practitioners find this test useful in corroborating the results of other testing methods.

Kinesiology

Kinesiology is an increasingly popular form of testing with practitioners and laypeople alike. There are different methods of kinesiology, but the one often employed in allergy/intolerance testing is known as 'muscle testing', in which the patient is examined for any changes to the normal resistance of a particular muscle group. The practitioner will begin by testing the resistance strength of the muscles. This can be done, for example, by pushing the patient's outstretched arm towards the ground. The substance being tested will then be placed in the patient's hand or mouth (without swallowing), or on another surface of the body. The practitioner then tests the muscle resistance again. The meaning of the result depends on the differences noticed by the practitioner. Anecdotal reports from many practitioners of applied kinesiology are very positive, but this method is probably a long way from being scientifically validated. Nevertheless, it may be of some use, probably depending greatly on the quality of the practitioner, and it is often inexpensive.

Skin Scratch/Skin Prick Tests

These tests are not the answer for everybody but they may be of reasonable value in measuring immediate reactions, especially to inhaled substances. To test for an immune-mediated inflammatory reaction, a sample of a suspected antigen is deposited just below the surface of the skin by placing a drop of the antigen solution on the skin and then inserting a needle just below the skin's surface. This is a sound premise because the release of inflammatory chemicals such as histamine is a typical antigenic occurrence. Regardless of the value of such tests, however, they are definitely low on the comfort scale!

CAUTION: If you suffer with severe airway constriction or other anaphylactic (severe, immediate) reactions upon ingestion of any foods, it is important to avoid any form of testing which requires actual ingestion of the foods in order to carry out the test. Severe asthmatics and others in this category should inform a qualified practitioner of their situation so that if a test is recommended, it will not be a potentially dangerous one.

CHAPTER 5

Treating Allergies

APPROACHES TO TREATMENT

Once you have successfully determined, one way or another, what you are allergic to, the next thing you will want to know is what you can do about it. The problem is that the treatment methods often used by the medical community are not suitable for dealing with much more than the symptoms themselves. Whether dealing with allergies from the orthodox or complementary perspective, the approach is of the utmost importance. If the approach is wrong or, as is usually the case, too narrow, then one cannot expect much long-term value, or to cease being allergic.

Suppressing the Symptoms

Understandably the first approach by the orthodox medical profession as well as many (but not all) natural practitioners is to deal with the prominent feature of the allergic reaction – the symptoms. This is a very important step for two main reasons:

TO TEMPORARILY REDUCE DISCOMFORT
The first priority of allergy sufferers is to feel better. Nobody could blame them for that, especially considering the often debilitating effect of many of the symp-

toms, such as violent sneezing attacks, blinding headaches, or embarrassing, unsightly skin rashes.

TO REDUCE POTENTIAL RISKS

For sufferers of anaphylactic (severe, immediate) reactions, such as severe breathing constrictions upon ingestion of any foods, suppressing the symptoms is the first priority. Although unusual, such situations can be life threatening. Everyone who falls into this classification should make sure that they have instant access to orthodox medication and medical assistance in the event of an attack *regardless of any personal preference for complementary therapies.*

Limitations to Treatment

Does it matter that most allergy sufferers receive therapy only for their symptoms, as these are what bother them most? The majority of sufferers do not realise that there is anything else that can be addressed. The truth is that there are significant limitations to this approach, including the following:

IGNORING THE ANTIGEN

The direct cause of any allergic reaction is the antigen itself. While some antigens, such as airborne pollens, simply cannot practically be avoided, most can, but only if the sufferer makes the effort to find out what he or she is allergic to, and to avoid future contact or ingestion. Suppressing the symptoms does not motivate the sufferer to concentrate on either identifying or avoiding the allergens.

Regardless of whether or not the symptoms are being suppressed, repeated contact with the antigen can be very damaging. First of all, the injury to the tissue of intestines, skin, respiratory tract, joints or any part that happens to be affected, can be made worse by chronic contact. Secondly, the immune system becomes less capable of dealing with destroying harmful bacteria, viruses and cancer cells due to the fact that it is constantly fighting large amounts of antigens. Chronic infections, such as those noted in the health disorder ME (myalgic encephalomyelitis) are common in long-term allergy sufferers.

IGNORING THE ALLERGIC TENDENCY

The idea of not trying to correct the sufferer's allergic tendency is particularly disturbing because this is the underlying factor in *all* cases of allergy. Avoiding the antigen is always the main priority in the short term, but in the long term, treating an allergic tendency will significantly reduce all existing allergies and their symptoms, as well as any that would otherwise have developed. Ideally, allergy sufferers would have their underlying tendency reduced, their antigens identified and their symptoms treated. In reality this rarely happens.

POTENTIAL SIDE-EFFECTS OF SYMPTOMATIC TREATMENTS

Treating the symptoms of an allergic reaction is often a useful step in a proper allergy programme, yet many treatments can have negative implications.

There are times when various symptoms of allergies are, for the most part, unreceptive to conventional treatments. A typical example of this is in the case of allergy-related depression. Certain antigens can cause changes in the brain 'environment', leading to depression or mood swings. In other cases, the depression might be an indirect symptom of malabsorption of certain nutrients responsible for correct brain chemistry. The typical drugs used for depression cannot untangle the mess created by antigenic chaos, nor can it replace nutrients required for proper brain chemistry. Any alleviation of symptoms would likely be minimal and temporary, and the treatment will often actually create further problems in an already confused chemical picture. Common treatments for the more tangible symptoms, such as eczema or perhaps asthma, often cause dependence or physiological damage to varying degrees.

COMMON MEDICAL TREATMENTS

Medical treatments for allergies, other than standard medication for individual symptoms, are limited. Treatments that address the allergy itself are widely available for hay fever, asthma, urticaria (hives) and reactions to insect bits and stings, but not for problems correlated to food allergies (although food allergies can sometimes cause anaphylactic reactions and asthma). It is worth looking briefly at what is available before discussing dietary alternatives in Chapter 5.

Antihistamines

Probably the most well-known common allergy treatment, antihistamines are the remedy of choice particularly in chronic and less severe cases of allergic inflammatory reactions. Histamine is one of the chemicals released by the mast cells which causes inflammation in conditions such as hay fever. Antihistamine drugs, such as terfenedine, temporarily reduce the release of histamine, which in turn temporarily reduces the respiratory symptoms. Such drugs do not reduce allergic tendencies, however, and repeated use can lead to side-effects. As airborne hay-fever allergens are not avoidable if you live in an area where they are plentiful, it is important to reduce both the hypersensitivity of the airways to the allergens and the overall allergic tendency in order to be less dependent on antihistamines. You might even opt for a natural agent which has antihistamine properties and few, if any, side-effects. (See sections on nutritional and herbal treatments, Chapter 5.)

Corticosteroids

The potent corticosteroids, called steroids for short, are another class of anti-inflammatory and anti-allergic drugs. Corticosteroids are actually chemicals which can be made by the body's adrenal glands. A certain class of corticosteroids, glucocorticosteroids, have effects which, among other things, reduce inflammation and allergic reactions, and suppress the immune system. At first glance these may seem wonderful for all allergy sufferers, but corticosteroids can be very dangerous and have significant side-effects even in their normal therapeutic dosage.

High-dose steroids can have damaging side-effects such as increased blood-sugar levels, poor immunity, bone degeneration, muscle wasting, fat deposition in the face and upper back, mood swings, fluid retention and associated weight gain, impotence, menstrual problems, high blood pressure, thinning of the skin and actual shrinkage of the adrenal glands leading to adrenal atrophy. In recent years efforts have been made to reduce these side-effects by encouraging local application of medication. Instead of taking a tablet for asthma, for example, an inhaler could be used instead, and a hydrocortisone cream could be used for inflammatory skin rash. Eventually, however, side-effects and dependency may well still occur, although often in a more local manner. And no matter how effective corticosteroids can be in treating particular symptoms, they will never correct or cure the actual condition which caused the symptom in the first place.

> **PLEASE NOTE:** If you have been prescribed corticosteroids of any type for asthma or an anaphylactic reaction, it could be dangerous for you to discontinue the medication without your doctor's consent and supervision.

Sodium Cromoglycate

Another anti-allergic drug used by the orthodox medical field, sodium cromoglycate is known as a mast-cell stabiliser. This is because it stabilises the surfaces of the mast cells and thus reduces the release of inflammatory chemicals such as histamine which would otherwise be triggered by the antibody response to the allergen. Although most often used for treating asthma in the form of an inhaler, it is also used for hay fever and inflammatory bowel disorders among other things. It appears to be more effective in treating asthmatic children than adults, and as it is not thought to be effective after the allergic reaction has occurred, it is used

> **PLEASE NOTE:** Any drug prescribed for severe asthma or other severe allergic reactions should not be discontinued without the consent and supervision of the doctor. Sudden discontinuation of certain anti-allergic drugs can induce a severe attack, so please do not disregard this warning.

only to prevent attacks. Occasional side-effects include coughing, irritation in area of contact and, in rare cases, headaches, nausea and dizziness.

NEGATIVE FOODS

In school we all learn a few basic aspects of nutrition, such as the four food groups, but this does not really stand us in good stead when dealing with food allergies, either our own or those of our children. Many important factors are left untold such as:

- whether the nutrients in the foods are likely to be absorbed
- whether the foods contain inherently harmful characteristics
- whether the foods contain elements likely to cause a reaction in susceptible people

There are many foods to which you may not be allergic that may aggravate your problem. The following information will outline which foods are most likely to be a problem in general for allergy sufferers, and why. It includes facts relevant to both ingestion allergies (foods) and respiratory allergies (hay fever and asthma).

Dairy Products
Even if you are not actually allergic to them, dairy products are one of the worst classes of food to consume if you have a tendency towards allergy-induced symptoms and disorders. Dairy products contain certain substances that make them perhaps the most common cause of food reactions such as allergies, intolerance, and chemical sensitivity.

CASEIN

Dairy products such as milk, cheese and yogurt contain casein, a protein difficult to break down, particularly if the digestive system is not functioning to capacity. Even those who are bolstering their digestive system may maintain a casein allergy, partly because excessive intestinal permeability may not yet have been corrected, as well as the fact that, even at the best of times, casein is difficult to digest completely. The more common symptoms associated with a dairy allergy (not to be confused with lactose intolerance) include:

- eczema
- catarrh and catarrhal deafness
- asthma
- migraine headache

LACTOSE INTOLERANCE

The most common symptoms associated with dairy products are probably caused by a lactose intolerance. Lactose is actually milk sugar. The body requires a special enzyme called lactase in order to break down lactose. If lactose is not broken down properly due to a lactase deficiency, it produces an intolerance reaction in the digestive system which ultimately leads to symptoms such as:

- abdominal bloating
- gas
- diarrhoea (sometimes violent)

Many people believe that we should not consume any dairy products after we are weaned from our mother's milk. They argue that no species other than humans seeks milk as a form of food beyond weaning, and particularly not milk from a different species. It is thought that this lack of affinity between humans and the milk of other species is manifested through allergy and/or intolerance. Children tend to have adequate amounts of the lactase enzyme while very young, but long before they reach 10 years of age, many no longer have the lactase content required to handle regular consumption of dairy products.

Goat's milk seems to be more similar to human milk than cow's milk, and many children seem to tolerate it better. Babies weaned from mother's milk directly on to goat's milk experience fewer problems, and goat's milk probably provides a more suitable balance of nutritional constituents than a typical milk substitute.

Lactose intolerance is particularly common in people of African, Asian, or Middle-Eastern origin, probably due to the traditionally low intake of milk products in their diet over the generations. It is thought that at least 75 per cent of such races are lactase-deficient, whereas this is the case for less than 20 per cent of those of northern European decent. Presumably it takes many generations for a particular population to adapt biochemically to severe changes in food intake.

FATS

Most dairy products contain significant amounts of arachidonic acid. This is an essential fatty acid, which means that the body needs it, but cannot manufacture it without a direct or indirect dietary supply. The primary function of arachidonic acid is to produce inflammatory chemicals such as leukotrienes and certain prostaglandins. Leukotrienes and their inflammatory counterpart histamine are released by the mast cells in order to cause inflammation at the site of an allergic reaction. Prostaglandins are hormone-like substances which mediate processes such as inflammation and blood-clotting. The prostaglandin which is involved in causing inflammation is prostaglandin E2 or PGE2. Arachidonic acid converts into PGE2, excesses of which are often considered a primary factor in an over-active inflammatory immune response. Nevertheless, there are ways to reduce one's tendency toward milk allergy and/or intolerance (see page 85).

Red Meat

Red meat is another type of food which can increase one's allergic tendency if consumed in large quantities. As with all foods, what is a small quantity for one person may be a large quantity to another.

FATS

Like dairy products, meat such as beef and pork contains large amounts of arachidonic acid, which can lead to a much higher tendency for excessive inflammatory reactions to occur. For both meat and dairy products, resultant chronic inflammatory reactions in locations such as the intestines and airways may exacerbate allergic tendencies, potentially creating another vicious circle.

DIGESTION

Meat has an extremely high protein content. Although meat protein is not one of the most common causes of allergies, it still can create a very basic problem.

Food-allergy sufferers tend to have much weaker digestion than those who are free of allergies. This is generally manifested in the incomplete digestion of proteins. Such people have difficulty digesting meat proteins. When meat is eaten with other protein foods, capacity to digest protein will be 'used up' to an extent on the meat protein, further compromising the ability to digest the non-meat protein. This concern can be avoided by not combining meat with any other form of protein in the same meal. In people with poor digestion, even if meat is eaten separately, however, the meat protein will not be amply digested either.

In these cases other problems arise which may increase food-allergy problems. Constipation or infrequent bowel movements can occur as the incompletely digested mass of meat slows the transit time of food through the intestines. As this gets worse, the meat can produce toxins that may irritate the walls of the intestinal tract. Chronic constipation may significantly harm the integrity of the bowel wall. Any toxins subsequently absorbed into the bloodstream have to be filtered by the liver, which reduces the liver's ability to filter out the undigested macro-nutrients, either from the meat or other foods which may absorb, thus enhancing the likelihood of larger amounts of circulating antigens. Also when meat proteins remain in the intestines for too long, certain bacteria begin to break down the protein constituents into polyamines (toxins linked to disorders such as psoriasis), and tyramine (a possible irritant in allergic migraine headaches).

To prevent such problems, it is generally best to reduce or eliminate the intake of all animal fats. The exception is the small amount of lean lamb meat allowable in the elimination diet. If you suffer from inhaled allergies such as hay fever, but not food allergies, it is still best to avoid meat and dairy products, at least partly because a great deal of inflammation is involved in both hay fever symptoms as well as asthma. Poultry (but not fatty duck or goose) can be used as a substitute for beef of pork. Many people have successfully substituted meat and dairy products with alternative substances for milk, cheese, and yogurt made from soybeans. This is not a bad idea at all, provided you are not allergic to soybeans!

Fried Food and Hydrogenated Fat

We have been led to believe that it is *always* healthier to use vegetable oils than animal fats, usually for reasons related to heart disease. This would be true if the oils were not used for high-temperature cooking methods such as frying. Vegetable-derived oils contain special fatty substances which are very important to our health. Unfortunately, they are also very unstable, chemically speaking. In other words, they are easily changed into a form which is no longer healthy, usually by heat and oxygen. The higher the heat, and the longer the exposure, the more unhealthy the oil becomes. You may have noticed that if you keep a bottle of vegetable oil too long, it begins to smell rancid. The rancidity is actually the process of the oxygen from the air changing the fats in the oil from healthy to unhealthy. The rancidifying process actually begins the minute the oil is exposed to air, and the longer the contact, particularly after opening a bottle, the more unhealthy the oil becomes. This process of the changing of oil due to heat or oxygen is called oxidation.

The oxidation of a fat produces 'free radicals', harmful molecules which travel through the body interrupting cellular processes, and eventually causing the cells to mutate or die. Free radicals are a primary factor in ageing, in many aspects of cardiovascular disease, cancer, arthritis, and other diseases. Oils cooked at a high temperature also increase inflammatory processes, and free radicals can cause untold damage to tissues such as those in the airways and the intestines. As a rule, it is fine, indeed beneficial, to use vegetable oils as long as they are raw. If you must cook with them, it is recommended that you do so at the lowest possible heat and for the shortest possible period of time.

What about margarine? As it is made with vegetable oil, you might reasonably assume that it is a healthy option, provided it is not used in cooking. Nothing could be further from the truth! The problem is that standard margarine is made from hydrogenated vegetable oil. Hydrogenation involves inundating the vegetable oil with hydrogen in a rather technical process and heating it to incredibly high temperatures. The end result gives margarine and other products such as vegetable shortening their spreadable characteristic. Unfortunately, it also makes them harmful – they increase biochemical processes that may lead to inflammation, heart disease and abnormal cell function.

Sugar

Sugar is an interesting dichotomy. On one hand, it represents much of what is bad in our diet, while on the other hand, it is one of the most essential components to life. Our body needs sugar for each cell to function, but the body has limitations on how fast it can utilise sugar's benefits. Complex carbohydrates such as whole-wheat, brown rice, or beans release sugars steadily. Refined sugars, such as ordinary white table sugar are more difficult for the body to deal with if taken in excess. As well as all the general problems associated with excessive sugar consumption, special problems exist where allergies are concerned.

Refined sugars cause a substantial release of the hormone adrenaline from the adrenal glands, which regulate stress reactions and inflammatory reactions. It is thought that this release of adrenaline sends the body into a stage similar to that of acute stress, when there is no need for such a release. Unfortunately, we are neither a 'bottomless pit' of adrenaline, nor can our adrenal glands easily withstand the constant stimulation which occurs with repeated high doses of stimulants such as sugar. This can have two consequences: the adrenals will be unable to become stimulated when necessary, leading to low stress tolerance, and/or the adrenals will fail to manufacture adrenaline quickly enough to compensate, thus leading to a lack of the hormone on demand. All efforts to keep the adrenals in good working order are vital. Avoiding the excessive intake of refined sugar is one way of preventing damaged adrenals.

There is another important link between refined sugar and allergies. Research in the United States has proved that white blood cells – which are responsible for killing antigens – are affected by the amount of refined sugar we eat. A couple of hours after eating refined sugar, the activity of certain white blood cells is drastically reduced. Shockingly, the research also showed that this was the case even when participants were given much less sugar than they usually consumed in an average day. As white blood cells are also vital for fighting life-threatening invaders such as cancer cells, harmful bacteria and viruses, imagine how significant a benefit could be brought about by a widespread reduction in sugar intake.

As far as allergies are concerned, immune and adrenal damaging agents such as refined sugar should be avoided, even in doses far below the average intake.

Caffeine

Caffeine, often found in tea, coffee, chocolate and certain soft drinks, can be a major contributor to allergic tendencies. Excessive consumption of caffeine has a similar effect on adrenal function as excessive amounts of sugar, in that both can cause unnecessary stimulation of adrenaline.

A stimulant drug, caffeine should be avoided in large quantities, even by healthy people. For someone with allergies, caffeine should probably be avoided completely unless it is being used medically*. Due to certain withdrawal-related effects, asthmatics should only eliminate caffeine slowly. If it is done too quickly, this causes a significant reduction in the level of adrenaline release that your body has become accustomed to.

Beverages containing caffeine also quickly drain certain nutrients from the body such as important B vitamins, and can inhibit the absorption of zinc, which is essential for strengthening the immune system, and iron.

Alcohol

In spite of its legal status, alcohol is still a potentially very harmful substance. It significantly reduces levels of most vitamins and several minerals, including many nutrients essential for the function of the immune system, stress control, allergy control and tissue repair. Alcohol, although it is not perceived as a stimulant (it

*Caffeine and a related substance called theophylline have been successfully used *in controlled medical dosage* for treatment of asthma. This is due to the fact that, if used properly, they can relax the bronchial tubes.

actually is a central nervous system depressant), does cause an initial rise in the release of adrenaline. The possible problems mentioned earlier, associated with this effect can be quite damaging from the standpoint of allergies.

The list of damaging effects of alcohol is quite lengthy. Alcohol consumption, especially in large quantities, may adversely affect bowel permeability and reduce the ability of the liver to filter antigens. Although there is a difference of opinion in terms of what constitutes 'excessive amounts', suffice it to say that allergy sufferers probably have a much lower tolerance for alcohol, not necessarily from the standpoint of getting drunk, but certainly in terms of many of the damaging effects listed above.

Tobacco

Many problems associated with smoking are well known. Among other things, smoking seriously damages the lungs and the entire respiratory tract. It may greatly increase the sensitivity of, or damage to, the tissue of the respiratory tract. This, as mentioned earlier, would increase the likelihood of antigen/antibody contact, possibility leading to asthma or hay fever.

Smoking may significantly compromise body stores of antioxidants (see page 68), and nicotine also causes substantial release of adrenaline.

The cynic would say that all this information on 'negative foods' adds credence to the saying 'if it tastes good or feels good, don't do it!' The allergy sufferer who has experienced the damaging effects of certain dietary and lifestyle habits would, however, say that it is not worth suffering for hours for something that gives you moments of pleasure. This is probably the best philosophy.

NATURAL TREATMENT OF SYMPTOMS AND ALLERGIC TENDENCY

There has been an enormous amount of research on how natural methods can positively affect allergic symptoms and those problems which may increase allergic tendencies. This information, which has been published in medical and scientific journals, outlines the proven beneficial effects of certain vitamins, minerals, enzymes, herbs and other natural substances. This section will explain how and why these work and show how they can be combined to create a research-based anti-allergy programme.

> **PLEASE NOTE:** As with all new health or medical regimes, it is important that you consult a qualified health practitioner before beginning your programme.

INHALED ALLERGENS

It is sometimes practically impossible to avoid the allergens responsible for problems such as hay fever and asthma, so it is essential to take all the safe and effective steps available to relieve the symptoms and the allergic tendency. If you are also allergic to things that cause symptoms other than respiratory reactions it would be enormously helpful to avoid those as well, as the more allergic reactions you sustain, the stronger your allergic tendency is liable to become.

This section looks at vitamins, minerals and herbs that can have a beneficial effect in the prevention and treatment of the symptoms of respiratory allergies, and on the allergic tendency itself. As well as the individual nutrients mentioned below, it is important not to neglect your basic need for necessary amounts of *all* essential vitamins, minerals and herbs. Many vitamins and minerals have a beneficial effect on asthma and hay fever. It may be advisable to consider using a multiple vitamin/mineral supplement.

Antioxidants

Antioxidants reduce the damaging effects of free radicals in the body (see pages 62–63). They may be of great value in the correction of:

- allergic symptoms (inflammation)
- antigen contact with antibodies (tissue weakness)
- slow removal of antibody/antigen complexes by immune cells
- thymus damage and the associated immune regulatory defects (see pages 13–14)

There are many antioxidants, including beta carotene, vitamins A, C, and E, and the minerals selenium and zinc. Besides the functions listed above, certain antioxidants may reduce the toxicity and damage caused by the more common inhaled irritants such as tobacco smoke, cleaning solvents, traffic pollution and paint fumes. All antioxidant nutrients will have general benefits in respiratory allergies and even non-allergic respiratory irritation and chemical sensitivity, and it is vital to make sure that the intake of these is adequate to meet such special needs. Some, such as vitamin C and beta carotene, are of particular importance in areas such as hay fever and asthma.

VITAMIN C

Vitamin C is perhaps the best known of the vitamins, and it is also one the most heavily researched. Also known as ascorbic acid, it is an essential vitamin, meaning we require it to live but the body cannot produce it without a dietary supply. Vitamin C can be effective in treating allergies, but only in higher dosages than are normally available in our diet, so supplementation may be required. Fortunately, like the other nutrients and herbs being discussed in this section, it is very safe, even at therapeutic levels.

As well as basic antioxidant properties, Vitamin C has a few different beneficial roles in respiratory reaction. It helps to quickly detoxify the body of histamine, which plays an enormous part in producing allergic inflammatory reactions. At certain levels vitamin C has been proven to help prevent asthmatic attacks in double-blind clinical trials*. To a great extent this is due to the fact that vitamin C prevents the constriction of the bronchial muscles. The antioxidant and histamine detoxification properties of the vitamin should be of value to people who suffer from hay fever, and those who suffer from asthma, whether caused by inhaled agents or foods.

Vitamin C is probably best known for its effect on strengthening of the immune system, hence its popular use for helping to relieve the common cold. This makes it of further value in reducing the immune weakness caused by chronic allergies.

*A double-blind trial is a scientific experiment using a testing substance and a placebo where neither the patient nor the person administering the test knows whether the patient is receiving the substance or the placebo. This effectively eliminates the 'placebo effect' and thus the test more accurately shows whether the people taking the tested substance fared better than those who actually received a placebo.

Less well known about this vitamin is its major role in the production of collagen, a necessary protein substance in the manufacture of the body's connective tissue. Collagen is a major component of the walls of the respiratory tract, thus improving collagen production is essential in repairing or preventing damage to the integrity of the tissue.

BETA CAROTENE

Carotenes are naturally occurring pigment agents found in plants and foods such as carrots, yellow vegetables and dark-green leafy vegetables. They may have significant preventive and symptomatic value in respiratory allergies, as well as protecting the body from certain after-effects of allergy-induced damage. Carotenes are some of the most powerful cell-protecting antioxidants known to man, and as a result they play a strong role as regulators of inflammation, and slow the process of tissue destruction. Certain carotenes, including beta carotene, are able to be converted into vitamin A in the liver. This conversion cannot lead to toxic amounts of vitamin A as the body only converts as much carotene as is needed at the time. Vitamin A is vital for proper maintenance of the respiratory tract and mucus membranes in general. The combination of the strong antioxidant effect and the vitamin A activity make substances such as beta carotene perhaps the most important for protecting and repairing the tissue which lines the respiratory walls. This could be very helpful in reducing the sensitivity of the walls to antigenic exposure.

Beta carotene can also help protect and enhance proper immune system function. This is due to its beneficial effect on the thymus gland, one of the main sites of the white blood cells which regulate immune reactions, such as T-helper cells and T-suppressor cells. These cells either encourage or discourage the attack of foreign invaders. A proper regulation of activity between these cells is vital, as it has been found that allergic individuals are often prone to excessive levels of helper T-cells compared to suppressor T-cells, hence far lower amounts of circulating antigens are needed to induce an immune-system attack.

Free-radical damage over time causes the thymus to shrink in size. This phenomenon causes the immune system to be less effective in killing viruses, cancer cells and harmful bacteria. This compounds the weakness created by the fact that the white blood cells are constantly having to attack antigens and are thus distracted from their main intended tasks. Beta carotene protects the thymus against shrinkage, thus producing a more suitable T-cell count, and also strengthening the protective effect of the immune system in general.

As with vitamin C, the therapeutic levels of Beta carotene may not be realistically obtainable through normal dietary intake. In spite of this, it is highly recommended to consume liberal amounts of foods containing beta carotene. Not only will even small amounts be better than nothing, there are also other valuable constituents to be found in such foods.

Magnesium

The mineral magnesium plays an essential role in the body. It is necessary, among other things, for the proper utilisation of calcium, healthy cardiovascular function, and basic nerve and muscle operation. In the prevention and treatment of asthma, it is the effect of magnesium on the muscles that is most relevant. Magnesium is necessary for the proper contraction and relaxation of muscles, and research has reported that it relaxes the smooth muscle of the bronchial tubes. Further studies have shown that magnesium successfully reduces attacks of bronchial asthma, presumably due to the relaxing effect on the bronchial muscle.

Although it appears that magnesium has no direct correlation to allergies in general, a magnesium deficiency may well make a sufferer more prone to asthmatic manifestation in the bronchial tubes. To avert the high risks involved in asthmatic reactions, everything possible should be done to reduce the susceptibility of the airways to spasm and constriction. Among other things, this would include:

- making sure magnesium intake was adequate (or therapeutic, if necessary)
- avoiding agents which drain magnesium from the body, such as alcohol and diuretics (but do not discontinue prescribed diuretics without the advice of a doctor)

Magnesium may not only reduce an asthma attack, it may also help to prevent attacks in the future. Although magnesium is a very safe nutrient, very high doses can cause diarrhoea.

Herbs

Nature has so much to offer to our health and well-being. Although valuable and important, technological advances in orthodox medicine have obscured many natural therapies that have been found safe and effective for hundreds, or even thousands, of years.

It would appear that at least part of the reason for the move away from nature in the past was the fact that the actions of many natural agents had not been put through tests which had been devised. This is definitely changing. Many of the natural agents have now been tested, and have proven to be effective and generally much safer than their orthodox medical counterparts. Often the effect of the natural agents is milder and slower than that of synthetic drugs, but sometimes it is actually stronger and faster, but still with many fewer or usually no side-effects at the necessary dosage.

Herbs represent the largest classification of natural agents that have been used for medicine throughout the world, and their use dates back thousands of years. Many of today's synthetic drugs are derived from herbs, although the synthetic refining of a particular active ingredient from a herb may produce side-effects which do not occur when the herb is taken by itself. Where hay fever and asthma are concerned, many herbs have substantial benefits when used properly in safely treating both the symptoms and the weakness or hyper-sensitivity of the respiratory tract.

SCUTELLARIA BAICALENSIS

Scutellaria is a Chinese herb which has recently been the subject of encouraging research. Although not widely used in western herbal medicine, it provides one of the most potent and beneficial actions in the treatment of allergic inflammatory reactions, and appears to be very safe to use.

Like many herbs, *Scutellaria* contains flavonoids. There are countless different flavonoids, each with individual pharmacological effects. The flavonoids in *Scutellaria baicalensis* are potent inhibitors of the release of inflammatory substances from the mast cells, including those known to be vastly more inflammatory and able to cause an allergic reaction than even histamine.

Many flavonoids possess strong antioxidant properties which counteract the negative effects of free radicals, such as tissue damage. The flavonoids in *Scutellaria* are no exception.

LIQUORICE ROOT

The herb liquorice root (also spelled licorice) has various remarkable properties. Traditionally, it was used primarily in Chinese medicine as an antidote to various toxins or poisons, and many such effects have subsequently been confirmed by scientific research.

Studies have also shown that liquorice contains substances that exhibit anti-inflammatory effects similar

---

PLEASE NOTE: If being prescribed corticosteroids, it would be advisable to tell your doctor if you are considering using liquorice root in case the dosage needs to be adjusted. In spite of the positive actions of liquorice root, there is one side-effect of corticosteroids that can also be a factor with liquorice root. Both corticosteroids and liquorice root cause potassium to be excreted from the body more quickly. This, over time, can lead to oedema and high blood pressure if potassium levels are not being compensated for through increased dietary intake or supplementation. If you use liquorice root over a longer period or in high doses for a moderate period, have your blood pressure checked occasionally and increase your potassium intake. Good sources are citrus fruit, bananas, fresh vegetables and baked potatoes. If you already suffer from high blood pressure, consult your doctor before using this herb and have your blood pressure checked frequently.

to those of corticosteroids (see page 55), albeit in a much milder way. Liquorice also increases the activity of the anti-allergic and anti-inflammatory substance cortisol. In theory, using liquorice should make corticosteroids more effective, probably at a lower dosage. It should also maximise the body's own production of corticosteroids. You may think that increasing the activity of corticosteroids may also increase their side-effects but remarkably quite the opposite is true. Among other things, liquorice root actually reverses certain damaging effects of corticosteroids, such as shrinkage of the thymus, a primary site of immune regulation. If used properly, liquorice root can be a valuable tool in the control of inflammatory allergic reactions, such as hay fever and asthma.

Quercetin

Quercetin is one of the most biologically active flavonoids. It can be found in onions, broccoli and red cherries, but for therapeutic levels it is often extracted from the herb *Sophora japonica*.

Research has proven that quercetin can significantly reduce or prevent many inflammatory processes that involve the mast cells, such as histamine release and leukotriene production. Quercetin is also an antioxidant, and increases the ability of the body to repair tissue by speeding collagen production. Its extraordinary biological activity, especially where allergic and inflammatory reactions are concerned, make quercetin a major priority in treatment and prevention of hay fever and asthma.

Treatment Programme

The following hypothetical programme uses medically

and scientifically researched substances for the natural treatment and prevention of respiratory allergies such as hay fever and asthma. This information is *not* intended to be prescriptive, and you should consult a qualified medical health practitioner before beginning any such programme. If you suffer from asthma caused by food allergies, it is recommended that you read the following section as it contains important information.

Avoid or reduce intake of:

- alcohol
- tobacco
- dairy products
- refined sugar
- caffeine (unless using medically)
- fried foods and hydrogenated fats (e.g. standard margarines)
- artificial preservatives (e.g. sulphites), colours (e.g. tartrazine) and flavours (e.g. monosodium glutamate-MSG)
- red meat (in excess)
- aspirin (unless prescribed – may cause asthma attacks in some)
- any foods to which you are allergic

Hypothetical recommendations (adult dosages):

- vitamin C (500–1,000 mg, 2–3 times daily)
- beta carotene (10–15 mg, 1–2 times daily)
- magnesium (as citrate or amino acid chelate, 150–200 mg, 1–2 times daily)
- scutellaria baicalensis (500–1,000 mg, 2–3 times daily)
- quercetin (200–500 mg, 2 times daily between meals)
- liquorice root (500–1,000 mg, 2 times daily, but do

not use liquorice root if you have high blood pressure without consulting your doctor; if using regularly, increase potassium intake)

Other important recommendations:

- antioxidant combination to be taken as directed on label
- multiple vitamin/mineral supplement with minimum 40–50 mg B-complex (to be taken as directed on label)

FOOD ALLERGIES

One of the major differences between food allergies and inhaled allergies is the fact that it is usually much easier to avoid an offending food once identified. The term 'easier' is used advisedly, as eliminating a food, especially one you love, is seldom easy. This section looks at substances that can have a beneficial effect in the prevention and treatment of the symptoms of food allergies, and on the allergic tendency itself.

Enzymes

Enzymes are involved in the breakdown or digestion of food components and are of key importance in the avoidance of antigenic activity. There are times when the availability of food-digesting enzymes is not even close to the level required by the body to deal with the food intake. Because protein, and to an extent, carbohydrate components are the main contributors in the development of food allergies, any way of ensuring their breakdown into free amino acids and simple sugars is to be highly recommended.

PANCREATIN

The pancreas secretes the enzymes protease, amylase and lipase, which break down protein, carbohydrates and fats respectively. They represent the final significant digestive action on proteins and carbohydrates, so they must be present in adequate quantities to meet the volume of food. This is often not the case, so supplementation (in the form of pancreatin) may be extremely useful in preventing incomplete digestion. Pancreatin splits protein chains into free amino acids, and carbohydrates into simpler sugars. It may represent one of the most important pieces in the puzzle of reducing the allergic tendency towards foods.

Pancreatin may also help reduce or eliminate non-allergic symptoms such as indigestion, heartburn, gas and abdominal bloating after meals. Because pancreatic lipase is hugely important in fat digestion, pancreatin may help those who do not tolerate fats very well.

HYDROCHLORIC ACID

Hydrochloric acid is a primary protein-digesting enzyme. Many people have too little to meet their volume of ingested protein, so ways of increasing this enzyme may need to be explored by the food-allergy sufferer. The mineral zinc and vitamin B6 are required for the body to produce adequate activity of hydrochloric acid, and increasing intake of those nutrients may have beneficial effects. Supplements of hydrochloric acid, in the form of betaine hydrochloride, should also be taken, at least at first, when meals containing protein are eaten.

Like pancreatin, hydrochloric acid may also be useful in reducing any related non-allergic symptoms, such as bloating, gas, heartburn and indigestion. Hydrochloric acid supplementation should *not* be taken on an empty stomach or used in excessive amounts. If you experience an unusual feeling of warmth in your stomach after taking such a supplement, reduce the amount to a point where this does not occur. If you suffer from or are prone to stomach or duodenal ulcers, consult a doctor before taking hydrochloric acid.

Quercetin

Quercetin, among the most biologically active flavonoids (see page 74) stabilises the surfaces of the mast cells, thereby inhibiting the release of histamine and the production of other inflammatory chemicals, such as leukotrienes. The effects achieved by these actions and the apparent safety of the substance makes quercetin an attractive tool in the prevention of allergic symptoms. Other benefits include the encouragement of tissue-protecting collagen production and antioxidant capabilities.

Antioxidants

See the section on antioxidants and respiratory allergies (page 68). The antioxidants of particular importance in food allergies include vitamins A and C, and zinc.

VITAMIN C

Vitamin C is beneficial in food allergies for some of the same reasons as it is so important in inhaled or respiratory allergies (see page 69). Although the prevention of bronchial muscle constriction (as seen when vitamin C is used therapeutically in asthma) may seem irrelevant to a food-allergy discussion, it must be remembered that one of the main causes of asthma attacks is allergies to various foods. Even if your food allergies do not result in asthma, vitamin C has vital properties: histamine-detoxifying effects, antioxidant activity and collagen-stabilising ability. Histamine is involved in the mechanical cause of many food-allergy reactions. As a result, any efforts to detoxify the body of residual histamine would be very useful in curtailing the inflammatory damage in the site of the reaction. As an antioxidant, vitamin C can help protect against tissue damage and certain inflammatory processes caused by free radicals. Collagen production is a major function of vitamin C. This is quite useful in the protection and repair or healing of the connective tissue of the intestinal walls. Vitamin C is also beneficial to the immune system.

PLEASE NOTE: Very large doses of vitamin C can cause temporary diarrhoea. This is not a cause for alarm, merely a gauge that tells you to reduce the dosage to the point where the diarrhoea does not persist. Nevertheless, diarrhoea is not conducive to a successful food-allergy treatment programme; nor does it help you assess your progress as you may be inclined to blame such an intestinal reaction on a food. The amounts of vitamin C recommended in cases of food or inhaled allergies is seldom at a dosage which would cause diarrhoea, but in certain individuals these doses can still produce loose stools. The benefits of vitamin C far outweigh any problems, but a recommended option, at least in food allergies, is a specially manufactured vitamin C with as close to a neutral pH as possible. Often called 'buffered' vitamin C, it is less likely to cause diarrhoea.

VITAMIN A

Vitamin A is essential for the proper health of the mucus membrane, a tissue which lines areas of the body where mucus is produced. Both the intestinal and respiratory tract are examples of these areas, hence the importance of this essential nutrient in the allergic disorders being discussed. In the case of food allergies, where the major mucus-producing tissues being addressed are in the intestines, vitamin A appears to be particularly vital. One type of immunoglobulin (see page 32), IgA, actually helps to inhibit the passage of antigens through the intestinal barrier. Vitamin A seems to be able to increase IgA levels in the intestinal wall area.

As a rule, vitamins are very safe, with very little chance of toxicity. Vitamin A, however, has a higher toxicity than other vitamins. As a result, it is best not to exceed 25,000–30,000 IU on a daily basis for long periods unless consulting a doctor. Although doses many times this amount have been used safely for a period of months under doctor's supervision, tolerance varies greatly from person to person.

> **CAUTION:** Both pregnant women and those trying to get pregnant must receive advice from a doctor before using separate supplementation of vitamin A. Doses which would be safe for an adult woman under normal circumstances may not be safe for a foetus. As a result, intake must be adjusted accordingly.

ZINC

The essential mineral zinc plays an important part in dozens of bodily functions. It is amazing just how versatile this trace mineral is compared to other nutrients, especially considering it is found in relatively small quantities in the body. Its relevance to food allergies is also very diverse.

Zinc is one of the primary substances involved in regulating and improving immune function. It is needed in adequate amounts for thymus function, immune-related hormone production, white-blood cell production and activity, etc. As we have established, the regulation and strengthening of the immune system is essential for correcting not only immune hypersensitivity to antigens, but also weakened immunity caused by the excessive concentration of white blood cells on antigens.

Zinc is also necessary for the proper activity of the enzyme hydrochloric acid. Hydrochloric acid is the primary enzyme in the stomach for the digestion of proteins. If activity is weak, then larger amounts of incompletely digested proteins are likely to pose an antigenic problem in the intestinal tract.

B Vitamins

Vitamin B_6, like zinc, is involved in several bodily functions, and is important in the correction of food allergies. It helps ensure availability of hydrochloric acid in the stomach, and thus aids protein digestion. It is also necessary for stress reduction and the production of adrenal hormones, and plays a part in the immune system as well.

Research has shown that vitamin B_{12} suppresses certain immunoglobulin reactions related to asthma and urticaria (hives), both of which can easily be caused by a food allergy. Taken orally, B_{12} tends to be minimally absorbed unless it is in a form that does not require the digestive system, such as lozenges which dissolve under the tongue and absorb through the membranes in the mouth. This is the main reason why injection is often used for therapeutic use of this vitamin.

Pantothenic acid, also known as B_5, is one of the most essential nutrients in the production of adrenal hormones. As a result, it is often classed as the primary 'anti-stress nutrient'. Stress causes the digestive system to be temporarily weakened, thus increasing the risk of the presence of incompletely digested food components. For this reason, as well as others, any measures which reduce the frequency and/or severity of stress should be considered paramount.

Although there are times (such as in cases of urticaria) when certain B vitamins may be needed in very high dosage, a B-complex supplement containing all the B vitamins will suffice for most people, provided that other steps are being taken.

Fibre

Dietary fibre plays a well-documented role in health, relieving constipation and reducing the risk of other colon-related disorders. There are actually several different types of fibre. The two types of most relevance to food allergies are insoluble and soluble fibre.

INSOLUBLE FIBRE

Insoluble fibre (e.g. cellulose) has the characteristic of not really changing consistency when exposed to water. Perhaps the classic example of insoluble dietary fibre is wheat bran. The term 'bran' refers to the outer coating of a grain. Wheat bran, sometimes considered by sceptics to be like 'glorified sawdust', does have health-giving properties; it speeds up the transit time of food waste through the intestines, and leads to production of important short-chain fatty acids. This improved transit time accounts to a great extent for its value in correcting constipation and possibly reducing the risk of diseases of the colon. It also helps remove waste residue which can be harmful to the intestinal walls.

The problem with insoluble fibre, especially wheat bran, is that wheat is a highly antigenic food, excessive intake of wheat bran may exacerbate diarrhoea, especially over a period of time, and excessive intake of wheat bran may bind with and reduce absorption of essential minerals.

SOLUBLE FIBRE

Soluble fibre is a different story altogether. When exposed to water, it softens and swells as it absorbs the water. Some more common sources of soluble fibre include oat bran, apple pectin and psyllium seed husks. Soluble fibre has intestinal cleansing properties, as does insoluble fibre; but instead of remaining coarse, soluble fibre is actually soft and soothing to the intestinal wall.

As far as food allergies are concerned, an increased intake of soluble fibre is highly recommended. Not only will it help remove faecal matter and residue that otherwise may lead to tissue-damaging toxins, but it can also help eliminate antigens before they create problems at the intestinal barrier. Furthermore, it can help correct constipation *and* diarrhoea. It may seem strange that the same substance can accomplish what appear to be opposite roles, but this is one of the other advantages of soluble fibre over insoluble fibre. As mentioned earlier, chronic diarrhoea is not only a common symptom of food allergies and intolerance; it is also a common cause of increased bowel permeability.

As oats are relatively high on the allergic scale, it is probably best to utilise the other forms of this type of fibre, such as psyllium seed husks.

Lactobacillus Acidophilus and Bifidobacterium

Although we tend to think of bacteria in negative terms, there are certain strains of bacteria that are very important in sustaining *healthy* human functioning. Perhaps the best examples of this are the beneficial intestinal bacteria such as lactobacillus acidophilus and bifidobacterium.

These bacterial strains, which are normal residents of our intestines, help maintain the proper environment in the intestinal tract. This includes controlling harmful bacterial growth, preventing overgrowth of the potentially damaging yeast *Candida albicans*, and promoting further digestion of sugars such as lactose (which commonly causes food intolerance to milk products).

The improved control of the intestinal environment reduces the risk of bowel damage and the associated permeability. Lactobacillus acidophilus may help to combat chronic diarrhoea and thus any diarrhoea-related intestinal damage, and it may reduce bowel damage caused by bacterial toxins.

Treatment Programme

The following hypothetical programme uses medically and scientifically researched substances for the natural treatment and prevention of food allergies and their symptoms. This information is *not* intended to be prescriptive, and you should consult a qualified medical health practitioner before beginning any such programme.

Avoid or reduce intake of:

- any food to which you are allergic
- alcohol

- dairy products (even if you are not allergic to them)
- refined sugar
- caffeine
- tobacco
- fried foods and hydrogenated fats (e.g. standard margarines)
- artificial preservatives (i.e. sulphites), colours (i.e. tartrazine), and flavours (e.g. monosodium glutamate – MSG)
- red meat (in excess)

Hypothetical recommendations (adult dosages):

- pancreatin (4x) (500–1,500 mg, during or immediately after major meals)
- betaine hydrochloride (300–600 mg, during or immediately after major meals, but do *not* use if prone to stomach or duodenal ulcers without first consulting a doctor, and reduce dosage if any unusual warmth is experienced in the stomach after taking)
- quercetin (200–500 mg, 2 times daily between meals)
- psyllium seed husks (1,000–3,000 mg, 1–2 times daily between meals with a full glass of water)
- vitamin C, preferably buffered (500–1,000 mg, 2–3 times daily)
- vitamin A (7,500 IU–10,000 IU, 1–2 times daily, but *not* if pregnant without medical advice)
- lactobacillus acidophilus (200–400 million organisms once daily – may contain other beneficial strains)
- multiple vitamin/mineral (with minimum 40–50 mg B-complex to be taken as directed on label)

Other important recommendations:

- zinc as picolinate or amino acid chelate (20–25 mg once daily)
- antioxidant combination (to be taken as directed on label)

BIBLIOGRAPHY

Atherton, D. *et al*, 'A double-blind controlled crossover study of an antigen avoidance diet in atopic eczema', *Lancet*, i, 1978, p. 401.

British Medical Association – Guide to Medicines and Drugs, Dorling Kindersley, London, 1991.

Brown, E. and Ruskin, S. 'The use of cevitaminic acid in the symptomatic and coseasonal treatment of pollinosos', *Annals of Allergy*, 7, 1949, pp. 65–70.

Buckley, R. 'Food allergy', *Journal of the American Medical Association*, 248, 1982, p. 2,627.

Clemenson, C. 'Histamine and ascorbic acid in human blood', *Journal of Nutrition*, 110, 4, 1980, pp. 662–8.

Coca, A. 'Art of investigating pulse diet record in familial non-reagenic food allergy', *Annals of Allergy*, 2, 1944, p. 1.

Commings, W. and Williams, E. 'Transport of large breakdown products of dietary protein through the gut wall', *Gut*, 19, 1978, p. 715.

De Weck, A.L. 'Pathophysiologic mechanisms of allergic and pseudo-allergic reactions to foods, food additives and drugs', *Annals of Allergy*, 53, 1984, pp. 583–6.

Dockhorn, R. and Smith, T. 'Use of chemically defined hypo-allergenic diet in the management of patients with suspected food allergy', *Annals of Allergy*, 47, 1981, pp. 264–6.

Finn, R. *et al*. 'Expanding horizons of allergy and the

total allergy syndrome',
Clinical Ecology, 3, 3, 1985,
pp. 129–31.

Foreman, J. (ed.) 'Mast cells
and the actions of
flavonoids', *Journal of
Allergy and Clinical
Immunology*, 73, 1984,
pp. 769–74.

Gerrard, J. *et al*, 'Familial
incidence of allergic
disease', *Annals of Allergy*,
36, 1976, p. 10.

Grosch, W. and Laskawy, G.
'Co-oxidation of carotenes
requires one soybean
lipoxygenase isoenzyme',
Biochem. Biophys. ACTA,
575, 1979, pp. 439–45.

Hikino, H. *Economic and
Medicinal Plant Research*,
vol. 1, Academic Press,
1985.

*Immunology and Clinical
Practice* 6, 1984, p. 123.

Innerfield, I. *Enzymes in
Clinical Medicine*, McGraw
Hill, New York, 1960.

Kamimura, M. 'Anti-inflammatory activity of vitamin
E', *Journal of Vitaminology*,
18, 4, 1972, p. 204.

Kimura, Y. *et al.* 'Studies on
scutellaria radix. VIII.
Effects of various
flavonoids on arachidonate

metabolism in leukocytes',
Planta Medica, 54, 1985,
pp. 132–6.

King, D.S. 'Can allergic exposure provoke psychological
symptoms? A double-blind
test' *Biol. Psychiatry*, 16, 1,
1981, pp. 3–19.

Kubo, M. *et al.* 'Studies on
scutellaria radix. VII. Anti-
arthritic and anti-inflammatory actions of
methanolic extract and
flavonoid components
from scutellaria radix',
Chem. Pharm. Bulletin, 32,
1984, pp. 2,724–9.

Lake, A. *et al.* 'Intestinal
goblet cell mucous release',
Journal of Immunology, 122,
1979, p. 834.

Lee, C. *et al*, 'Provocative
testing and treatment for
foods', *Archives of
Otolaryngology*, 90, 1969,
p. 113.

Mansfield, L.E. *et al*, 'Food
allergy and adult migraine:
Double-blind and mediator
confirmation of an allergic
etiology', *Annals of Allergy*,
55, 1985, p. 126.

McCarty, M. 'Can dietary
selenium reduce
leukotriene production?',
Medical Hypothesis, 13,

1984, pp. 45–50.

McGovern J.J. 'Corrlation of clinical food allergy symptoms with serial pharmacological and immunological changes in the patient's plasma', *Annals of Allergy*, 44, 1980, p. 57.

Middleton, E. and Drzewiecki, G. 'Naturally occurring bioflavonoids and human basophil histamine release', International Archives of Allergy and Applied Immunology, 77, 1985, pp. 155–7.

Murray, M. and Pizzorno, J. *Encyclopaedia of Natural Medicine*, Macdonald and Co., London, 1990.

Nasr, S. *et al.* 'Concordance of atopic and affective disorders', *Journal of Affective Disease*, 3, 1981, p. 291.

Nutrition Foundation, *Present Knowledge in Nutrition*, fifth edition, Washington, DC, 1984.

Ogle, K. and Bullocks, J. 'Children with allergic rhinitis and/or bronchial asthma treated with elimination diet: a five year follow-up', *Annals of Allergy*, 44, 1980, pp. 273–8.

Paganelli, R. *et al.* 'Detection of specific antigen within circulating immune complexes', *Lancet*, i, 1979, p. 1,270.

Parish, P. *Medical Treatments: the Benefits and Risks*, Penguin, 1991.

Passmore, R. and Eastwood, M. *Human Nutrition and Dietetics*, Churchill Livingstone, Edinburgh, 1986.

Pearce, F. *et al. Journal of Allergy and Clinical Immunology*, 73, 1984, pp. 819–23.

Pekarek, R. *et al.* 'Abnormal cellular immune responses during acquired zinc deficiency', *American Journal of Clinical Nutrition*, 32, 1979, p. 1,466.

Peliken, Z. *et al.* 'Bronchial asthma due to food allergy', XII International Congress of Allergy and Clinical Immunology, Oct. 1985, Washington, DC.

Podell, R. 'Food allergy: A mainstream perspective', *Clinical Ecology*, 3, 2, 1985, pp. 79–84.

Ransberger, K. 'Enzyme treatment of immune complex diseases', *Arthritis and Rheumatism*, 8, 1986, pp. 16–19.

Reinhardt, M.C. 'Macromolecular absorption of food antigens in health and disease', *Journal of Allergy*, 53, 1984, p. 597.

Rinkel, H. *et al*, 'The diagnosis of food allergy', *Archives of Otolaryngology*, 79, 1964, p. 71.

Rinkel, H. 'Food allergy IV. The function and clinical application of the rotary diversified diet', *Journal of Pediatrics*, 32, 1948, p. 266.

Rowe, A.H. and Rowe, A. *Food Allergy – Its Manifestation and Control and the Elimination Diets*, C.C. Thomas, Springfield, Illinois, 1972.

Sampson, H. 'Role of immediate food hypersensitivity in the pathogenesis of atopic dermatitis', *Journal of Allergy and Clinical Immunology*, 71, 1983, pp. 473–80.

Schauff, C. *et al. Human Physiology*, Time Mirror/Mosby College, St Louis, Mo., 1990.

Segal, R. *et al. Journal of Pharmaceutical Science*, 74, 1, 1985, p. 79.

Tan, Y. and Collins-Williams, C. 'Aspirin-induced asthma in children', *Annals of Allergy*, 48, 1982, pp. 1–5.

Trevino R.J. 'Immunologic mechanisms in the production of food sensitivities', *Laryngoscope*, 91, 1981, p. 1,913.

Voet, D. and Voet, J. *Biochemistry*, John Wiley & Sons, New York, 1990.

Werbach, M. *Nutritional Influences on Illness*, Thorsons, London, 1987.

Yashimoto, T. *et al.* 'Flavonoids: Potent inhibitors of arachidonate 5-lipoxygenase', *Biochem. Biophys. Res. Commun.*, 116, 1983, pp. 612–18.